Occupational
and Physical Therapy
in Educational Environments

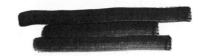

Occupational
and Physical Therapy
in Educational
Environments

Irene R. McEwen
Editor

The Haworth Press, Inc.
New York • London

Occupational and Physical Therapy in Educational Environments has also been published as *Physical & Occupational Therapy in Pediatrics*, Volume 15, Number 2 1995.

The development, preparation, and publication of this work has been undertaken with great care. However, the publisher, employees, editors, and agents of The Haworth Press and all imprints of The Haworth Press, Inc., including The Haworth Medical Press and Pharmaceutical Products Press, are not responsible for any errors contained herein or for consequences that may ensue from use of materials or information contained in this work. Opinions expressed by the author(s) are not necessarily those of The Haworth Press, Inc.

The Haworth Press, Inc., 10 Alice Street, Binghamton, NY 13904-1580 USA

Library of Congress Cataloging-in-Publication Data

Occupational and physical therapy in educational environments / Irene R. McEwen, editor.
    p. cm.
    "Occupational and physical therapy in educational environments has also been published as Physical & occupational therapy in pediatrics, volume 15, number 2, 1995"–t.p. verso.
    Includes bibliographical references.
    ISBN 1-56024-777-0 (alk. paper)
    1. Physical therapy for children–United States. 2. Occupational therapy for children –United States. 3. Handicapped children–Education–United States. I. McEwen, Irene R. II. Physical & occupational therapy in pediatrics.
LB3458.033 1995
615.8'2'0834–dc20
                                                                95-42894
                                                                  CIP

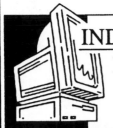

INDEXING & ABSTRACTING

Contributions to this publication are selectively indexed or abstracted in print, electronic, online, or CD-ROM version(s) of the reference tools and information services listed below. This list is current as of the copyright date of this publication. See the end of this section for additional notes.

- *Academic Abstracts/CD-ROM,* EBSCO Publishing, P.O. Box 2250, Peabody, MA 01960-7250

- *Biosciences Information Service of Biological Abstracts (BIOSIS),* Biosciences Information Service, 2100 Arch Street, Philadelphia, PA 19103-1399

- *Child Development Abstracts & Bibliography,* University of Kansas, 2 Bailey Hall, Lawrence, KS 66045

- *CINAHL (Cumulative Index to Nursing & Allied Health Literature), in print, also on CD-ROM from CD PLUS, EBSCO, and SilverPlatter, and online from CDP Online (formerly BRS), Data-Star, and PaperChase. (Support materials include Subject Heading List, Database Search Guide, and instructional video),* CINAHL Information Systems, P.O. Box 871/1509 Wilson Terrace, Glendale, CA 91209-0871

- *Developmental Medicine & Child Neurology,* Mac Keith Press, 526-529 High Holborn House, 52-54 High Holborn, London WC1V 6RL, England

- *Exceptional Child Education Resources (ECER), (online through DIALOG and hard copy),* The Council for Exceptional Children, 1920 Association Drive, Reston, VA 22091

- *Excerpta Medica/Secondary Publishing Division,* Elsevier Science Inc., Secondary Publishing Division, 655 Avenue of the Americas, New York, NY 10010

- *Health Source: Indexing & Abstracting of 160 Selected health related journals, updated monthly:* EBSCO Publishing, 83 Pine Street, Peabody, MA 01960

(continued)

- *Health Source Plus: expanded version of "Health Source" to be released shortly:* EBSCO Publishing, 83 Pine Street, Peabody, MA 01960

- *INTERNET ACCESS (& additional networks) Bulletin Board for Libraries ("BUBL"), coverage of information resources on INTERNET, JANET, and other networks.*
  - JANET X.29: UK.AC.BATH.BUBL or 00006012101300
  - TELNET: BUBL.BATH.AC.UK or 138.38.32.45 login 'bubl'
  - Gopher: BUBL.BATH.AC.UK (138.32.32.45). Port 7070
  - World Wide Web: http://www.bubl.bath.ac.uk./BUBL/home.html
  - NISSWAIS: telnetniss.ac.uk (for the NISS gateway)
  The Andersonian Library, Curran Building, 101 St. James Road, Glasgow G4 ONS, Scotland

- *Inventory of Marriage and Family Literature (online and CD/ROM),* Peters Technology Transfer, 306 East Baltimore Pike, 2nd Floor, Media, PA 19063

- *Occupational Therapy Database (OTDBASE),* 3485 Point Grey Road, Vancouver, BC V6R 1A6, Canada

- *Occupational Therapy Index,* British Library Medical Information Service, Boston Spa, Wetherby, West Yorkshire, LS23 7BQ, United Kingdom

- *OT BibSys,* American Occupational Therapy Foundation, P.O. Box 31220, Rockville, MD 20849-1220

- *Social Work Abstracts,* National Association of Social Workers, 750 First Street NW, 8th Floor, Washington, DC 20002

- *Sport Database/Discus,* Sport Information Resource Center, 1600 James Naismith Drive, Suite 107, Gloucester, Ontario K1B 5N4, Canada

- *Violence and Abuse Abstracts: A Review of Current Literature on Interpersonal Violence (VAA),* Sage Publications, Inc., 2455 Teller Road, Newbury Park, CA 91320

(continued)

SPECIAL BIBLIOGRAPHIC NOTES

related to special journal issues (separates)
and indexing/abstracting

- [ ] indexing/abstracting services in this list will also cover material in any "separate" that is co-published simultaneously with Haworth's special thematic journal issue or DocuSerial. Indexing/abstracting usually covers material at the article/chapter level.

- [ ] monographic co-editions are intended for either non-subscribers or libraries which intend to purchase a second copy for their circulating collections.

- [ ] monographic co-editions are reported to all jobbers/wholesalers/approval plans. The source journal is listed as the "series" to assist the prevention of duplicate purchasing in the same manner utilized for books-in-series.

- [ ] to facilitate user/access services all indexing/abstracting services are encouraged to utilize the co-indexing entry note indicated at the bottom of the first page of each article/chapter/contribution.

- [ ] this is intended to assist a library user of any reference tool (whether print, electronic, online, or CD-ROM) to locate the monographic version if the library has purchased this version but not a subscription to the source journal.

- [ ] individual articles/chapters in any Haworth publication are also available through the Haworth Document Delivery Services (HDDS).

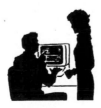

Occupational and Physical Therapy in Educational Environments

CONTENTS

ABOUT THE EDITOR

Irene R. McEwen, PhD, is Associate Professor of Physical Therapy at the University of Oklahoma Health Sciences Center in Oklahoma City. She is a consultant and expert witness for the Special Litigation Section, Civil Rights Division, of the U.S. Department of Justice and is a member of the Committee on Increasing Providers of Services, Oklahoma Commission on Child and Youth Interagency Coordinating Council for Special Services to Children and Youth. Dr. McEwen is a board certified clinical specialist in pediatric physical therapy with the American Board of Physical Therapy Specialties. Her professional activities include the Board of Directors, United States Society for Augmentative and Alternative Communication; the Pediatric Specialty Council of the American Board of Physical Therapy Specialties; the Education Committee, Section of Pediatrics, of the American Physical Therapy Association; and the Board of Directors, Oklahoma Society for Augmentative and Alternative Communication.

Introduction

Irene R. McEwen

When Public Law 94-142 was enacted by Congress in 1975, it mandated that related services, including occupational therapy and physical therapy, be provided "as may be required by a handicapped child to benefit from special education."[1] Over the nearly 20 years since the law was implemented, public schools have become the most common practice setting of occupational therapists and physical therapists who work with children.[2,3] In the professions as a whole, approximately 18% of occupational therapists and 4.6% of physical therapists provide services for children with disabilities in public school programs.

Although the law increased availability of special education and related services for students with disabilities, the required link between therapy and benefit from special education led to confusion and controversy about who should receive therapy, the purposes of therapy, and how services should be provided. Although the role of school-based therapy has been clarified somewhat since 1975, concerns remain, not only among therapists, but among parents, administrators, and legislators.

The foundation for school-based therapy services is a good understanding of the laws and regulations that guide special education programs. Yet, many therapists have limited knowledge of them.[3] Mary Jane Rapport's article in this volume, "Laws that Shape Therapy Services in Educational Environments," summarizes the major statutory law, federal regulations, and case law interpretation in which school-based practice is grounded. Therapists who have a firm grasp on this information and related state

Irene R. McEwen, PhD, PT, PCS, is Associate Professor, Department of Physical Therapy, University of Oklahoma Health Sciences Center, P.O. Box 26901, Oklahoma City, OK 73190.

[Haworth co-indexing entry note]: "Introduction." McEwen, Irene R. Co-published simultaneously in *Physical & Occupational Therapy in Pediatrics* (The Haworth Press, Inc.) Vol. 15, No. 2, 1995, pp. 1-3; and: *Occupational and Physical Therapy in Educational Environments* (ed: Irene R. McEwen) The Haworth Press, Inc., 1995, pp. 1-3. Single or multiple copies of this article are available from The Haworth Document Delivery Service [1-800-342-9678, 9:00 a.m - 5:00 p.m. (EST)].

regulations will have a good basis for making lawful and appropriate decisions that will stand up under administrative or due process scrutiny.

Working knowledge of current "best practices" in pediatric therapy is also necessary for making appropriate decisions in school-based practice. Contemporary theories of motor development, motor control, and motor learning have had a major impact on therapy for school age children with disabilities over the past five years, regardless of whether they receive therapy in school or in clinical settings. M'Lisa Shelden and I review some of the recent changes in our article, "Pediatric Therapy in the 1990s: The Demise of the Educational versus Medical Dichotomy."

How to decide which students should receive occupational therapy or physical therapy at school has been the subject of much debate. Since before Public Law 94-142 was implemented, therapists and other special education personnel have been trying to develop decision-making rules and tools to help them identify students who need school therapy services. Early criteria included age, severity of disability, and behavior; later decision-making tools used discrepancies between cognitive and motor skills or focused on access to materials and mobility.[4,5] Neither these nor most other criteria have survived clarification of lawful decision-making that meets the unique needs of students with disabilities. Michael Giangreco's article, "Related Services Decision-Making: Foundational Component of Effective Education for Students with Disabilities," describes a strong team approach to determining a student's need for related services, which takes into account the unique characteristics of both the student and the educational team.

Anita Bundy applies team decision-making and current practices to assessment and intervention in her article, "Assessment and Intervention in School-Based Practice: Answering Questions and Minimizing Discrepancies." The approach that she describes clearly illustrates a relationship between therapy and educational programs that results in meaningful outcomes for students.

Schools are not the only setting in which many students with disabilities receive services, so coordination among various medical, educational, and social agencies is essential to avoid gaps, overlaps, and cross purposes. Barrie O'Connor's qualitative study, "Challenges of Interagency Collaboration: Serving a Young Child with Severe Disabilities," reveals the difficult role a child's mother must play in coordinating programs and the problems that result when school-based therapists are unable to collaborate with personnel in other programs that a child attends. The author and the study are Australian, which may surprise some readers because the issues presented are so similar to those found in the United States.

As I write these comments in March 1995, the Individuals with Disabilities Education Act (IDEA) is before Congress for reauthorization and rumors are rampant that occupational therapy, physical therapy, and other related services may be eliminated from the law. Assuming we survive this time, we *must* more clearly define an appropriate role for therapists in the schools and we must provide services that have evident value if occupational therapy and physical therapy are to remain available to students with disabilities when IDEA is next reauthorized. The articles in this special volume are intended to assist therapists and other team members with this effort.

I sincerely thank the authors, not only for their fine work, but for their willingness to go through "just this one more little revision" and still meet the deadlines. I am also grateful to Suzann Campbell for the opportunity to bring together this collection of articles.

REFERENCES

1. Education for All Handicapped Children Act, Public Law 94-142. U.S. Congress, Senate, 94th Congress; 1995.

2. *1990 Member Data Survey.* Rockville, Md: American Occupational Therapy Association; 1991.

3. Sweeney JK, Heriza CB, Markowitz R. The changing profile of pediatric physical therapy: a 10-year analysis of clinical practice. *Pediatr Phys Ther.* 1994; 6: 113-118.

4. Chandler BE. Keeping occupied at school. *OT Week.* 1994; December 15: 24.

5. Taylor D, Christopher M, Freshman S, McEwen I. *Pediatric Screening: A Tool for Occupational and Physical Therapists* (2nd ed). Seattle, WA: University of Washington, Health Sciences Center for Educational Resources; 1983.

6. Carr SH. Louisiana's criteria of eligibility for occupational therapy services in the public school system. *Am J Occup Ther.* 1990; 44: 503-506.

Laws That Shape Therapy Services in Educational Environments

Mary Jane K. Rapport

SUMMARY. The delivery of physical therapy and occupational therapy in schools hinges, at least in part, on an accurate understanding of educational and civil rights laws that mandate services to children with disabilities in educational environments. Frequently, therapists, in addition to physicians, parents, school administrators, and teachers, have misconceptions regarding eligibility for therapy services provided at school district expense, the nature of therapy services in schools, and the frequency with which those services can and should be provided in educational environments. Most of the children who receive physical therapy, occupational therapy, or both in educational environments have disabilities that adversely affect their educational performance, and the assessments and interventions provided by therapists in educational environments are intended to be closely linked to the child's educational program. The legal information provided in the following paper summarizes the major provisions of statutory law, federal regulations, and case law interpretation that define the perimeters established, and continually redefined, for the delivery of physical therapy and occupational therapy in schools. *[Article copies available from The Haworth Document Delivery Service: 1-800-342-9678.]*

INTRODUCTION

A physical therapist or occupational therapist employed by a public school district may be faced with a service delivery decision similar to that

Mary Jane K. Rapport, PhD, PT, is Assistant Professor, Department of Special Education, College of Education, University of Florida, G315 Norman Hall, Gainesville, FL 32611.

[Haworth co-indexing entry note]: "Laws That Shape Therapy Services in Educational Environments." Rapport, Mary Jane K. Co-published simultaneously in *Physical & Occupational Therapy in Pediatrics* (The Haworth Press, Inc.) Vol. 15, No. 2, 1995, pp. 5-32; and: *Occupational and Physical Therapy in Educational Environments* (ed: Irene R. McEwen) The Haworth Press, Inc., 1995, pp. 5-32. Single or multiple copies of this article are available from The Haworth Document Delivery Service [1-800-342-9678, 9:00 a.m - 5:00 p.m. (EST)].

described in the following scenario: Douglas, an 8-year-old boy, was diagnosed with cerebral palsy at 4 months of age. He received numerous services as part of an early intervention program. Douglas is currently in the second grade at a local elementary school. He ambulates independently despite several observable gait deviations, and he tires more rapidly than his typically developing peers. He also has difficulty performing some of the more complex activities on the playground (e.g., climbing bars and tether ball). As a result of limited use of his left arm, Douglas requires modifications for many of the projects in art class. He is able to complete all assigned written seat work in academic subjects with either additional time or the use of a computer for word-processing. Should Douglas receive physical therapy, occupational therapy, or both at school district expense?

Several other pieces of information are necessary to answer this question. In Douglas' case, it is possible that the local school district may not be financially responsible for providing therapy for Douglas. This outcome, however, does not preclude the fact that Douglas might benefit from continued therapy provided in the community (i.e., therapy that is financed by resources other than the school district) to work on goals that are related to, but not directly assimilated into, his educational program. For example, Douglas may continue to work with a community-based therapist on skills that will eventually lead to improved or independent performance on various pieces of playground equipment. Although the ability to recreate independently may be an educationally-related goal for some children with disabilities, the ability to independently negotiate all pieces of playground equipment may not be a goal of educational relevance for Douglas. Age is but one factor that might be considered by a child's multidisciplinary team in determining the importance of providing therapy services related to the use of playground equipment. Conversely, the team may identify areas in which Douglas' disability does adversely affect his educational performance (e.g., high level of fatigue related to energy expenditure required to walk or limited use of his left arm for classroom activities) and may recommend therapeutic intervention as related services to be provided at school district expense. If Douglas' multidisciplinary team decides that he needs therapy to accomplish his educational goals, whatever they are, or to have access to or be maintained in the least restrictive educational environment, then the school district needs to provide it.

Understanding the role of occupational therapy and physical therapy in the educational environment has always been important, but in light of the current shortage of therapists and the mounting financial concerns of school districts nationwide, it has become ever more critical that therapy services be provided in accordance with both best practice and the parameters established by federal and state law. Appropriate delivery of therapy services in schools hinges, at least in part, on an accurate understanding of the laws that mandate related services for children with disabilities in educational environments.

STATUTES, REGULATIONS, AND CASE LAW

The provision of therapy services has been included in federal education statutes[1] and described briefly in accompanying federal regulations.[2] Statutes are legislative acts and regulations are the guidelines established by governmental agencies to carry out the laws or statutes. State statutes and regulations, as well as local board policies, provide additional guidelines for the delivery of therapy services in the educational environment. The federal component of this legal system provides the framework within which other jurisdictions must comply. As a result, neither state statutes nor local board policy may establish standards of service delivery below those set by federal statutes and regulations governing such practices. Figure 1 provides a visual representation of the legislative impact on the delivery of therapy services.

Statutes, the formal legislative component of the law, are developed and approved when sufficient case law and changing societal trends cause legislators to accept a "call" for action. It is through such legislative processes that updated federal and state statutes since the mid 1970s have included physical therapy and occupational therapy as related services to be provided at no cost to parents within the educational programs of children with disabilities. Federal regulations provide many general and specific guidelines for the delivery of services to children with disabilities, but state and local laws, board policies, and procedures also are important in determining eligibility and developing guidelines for the delivery of services. Case law, or judge-made law, provides additional information and interpretation of existing statutes and regulations when two parties have disagreed on the legal interpretation of a rule, regulation, or policy and have brought the disagreement before the courts. When considering the case study of Douglas described above, the provision of therapy services would be based not only on federal and state statutes (laws) and regulations (rules and procedures) but also on local board policy and perhaps on interpretation from a state hearing officer in response to due process or an otherwise judicially-based decision.

The legislative "hierarchy" represented in Figure 1 depicts federal

FIGURE 1. Legislative Impact on the Delivery of School-Based Therapy Services

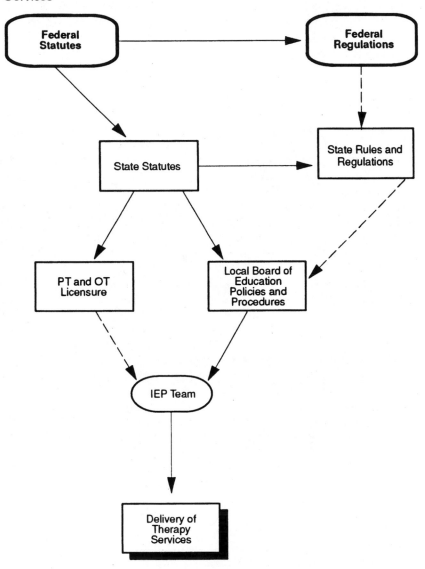

statutes as having precedence over state and local governments and agencies. This hierarchical structure also exists within the judicial system, whereby decisions conferred by the United States Supreme Court supersede all decisions made in any lower courts of law (e.g., state supreme courts, federal district courts, and federal appellate courts).

Several federal laws contain provisions for delivery of physical therapy and occupational therapy in schools. The most important of these is the Individuals with Disabilities Education Act (IDEA)[1] which requires compliance by all federal financial recipients in the provision of special education and related services to children who have disabilities that adversely affect educational performance. Section 504 of the Rehabilitation Act (RA)[3] and the Americans with Disabilities Act (ADA)[4] represent other important civil rights statutes that also affect the delivery of therapy services to children with disabilities in schools, although to a lesser degree than IDEA. These statutes, and their impact on therapy services in schools, will be described later. Figure 2 depicts how children with disabilities may be eligible for physical and/or occupational therapy services in schools according to the federal statutory definitions provided under the RA (Section 504), the ADA, and IDEA.

THE INDIVIDUALS WITH DISABILITIES EDUCATION ACT

Physical therapy and occupational therapy are included among the long list of related services in the Individuals with Disabilities Education Act of 1990 (formerly the Education of the Handicapped Act) that may be required "to assist a child with a disability to benefit from special education."[5] IDEA is the single most influential piece of federal legislation associated with the delivery of therapeutic intervention within educational environments. Two parts of the statute contain information specific to the delivery of physical therapy and occupational therapy: Part B[6] and Part H.[7] Part B currently applies to children ages 3 through 21 who require specially designed instruction to meet their unique needs.

Part H responds to the needs of children birth through age 2 (i.e., up to 36 months of age or the child's third birthday) who have an identified disability and who are experiencing, or have a high probability of experiencing, developmental delay and to their families.[8] Children who are at-risk for substantial developmental delay without early intervention are also included under Part H at the state's discretion.[9] Federal legislation mandating services to very young children (Title I: birth through age 2, and Title II: ages 3 through 5) with disabilities, and those who are at-risk, was implemented with the enactment of Public Law 99-457, the 1986

FIGURE 2. Statutory Eligibility for School-Based Therapy Services

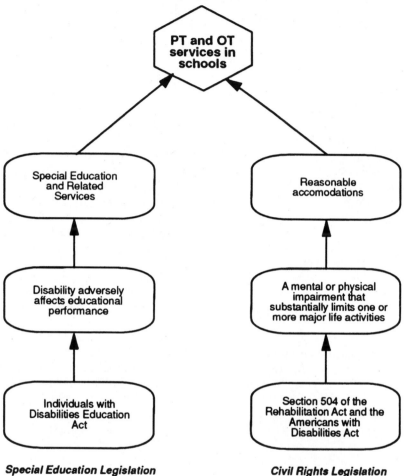

Amendments to the Education of the Handicapped Act (EHA).[10] Physical therapy and occupational therapy are provided as related services under Part B[5] and as early intervention services under Part H.[11]

Part B has a far greater impact than Part H on the delivery of therapy services in schools simply by virtue of the age range of children protected under this statute (ages 3 through 21), but Part H does provide services for young children in educationally-related, center-based locations when appropriate. Part H programs are under the auspices of the Department of Education in those states where that state department has been designated as the lead agency for early intervention services. This paper will focus primarily on Part B in Table 1, although the regulations for several relevant sections of Part H can be found in Table 2 and compared with the similar sections from Part B in Table 1. The tables provide definitions for several important terms used within IDEA pertaining to the delivery of special education and related services.

IDEA, like many other federal statutes, requires periodic reauthorization to assure continued appropriations and provide opportunities for modifications, additions, or deletions in the procedural and substantive components of the existing statute. As the reauthorization process that began last year (1994) continues in 1995 before the 104th Congress, it does not appear that there will be significant changes affecting the delivery of physical therapy and occupational therapy as related services in schools.

Due Process

IDEA not only provides financial support to school districts, albeit a minimal contribution, for special education and related services (including physical therapy and occupational therapy) for eligible children with disabilities, but also guarantees the rights of due process to children with disabilities and their parents/guardians. Due process procedure provides an avenue for recourse should parents feel that their child's educational rights have been violated. Figure 3 identifies the steps that might follow a disparity between two parties (i.e., parents and school district) on either a procedural or a substantive issue resulting in the initiation of due process under IDEA. Procedural issues stem from the failure to follow proper procedure as defined under IDEA (e.g., failure to notify parents prior to a change in placement); substantive issues involve claims that are related to the content and delivery of the child's educational program (e.g., lack of agreement on the amount or nature of therapy services).

Due process begins with a formal response to a complaint through an administrative review at the school district level and may include mediation at some point following the review in an attempt for the parties to reach resolution. When either party, be it parent or school district, continues to be dissatisfied, the next step in due process involves a hearing before an independent hearing officer in those states operating a two-tier system. In single-tier states, there is no intermediary step (independent hearing officer), and continuing disparities are heard before a state-level hearing officer. Should the disagreement fail to be resolved at local and

TABLE 1. Definitions from the Individuals with Disabilities Education Act (IDEA)–Part B

Term	Definition	Citation – Code of Federal Regulations
Special Education	Specially designed instruction, at no cost to the parents, to meet the unique needs of a child with a disability.	34 C.F.R. § 300.17(a)(1)
Related Services	Transportation and such developmental, corrective, and other supportive services as are required to assist a child with a disability to benefit from special education, and includes speech pathology and audiology, psychological services, physical and occupational therapy, recreation, including therapeutic recreation, early identification and assessment of disabilities in children, counseling services, including rehabilitation counseling, and medical services for diagnostic or evaluation purposes. The term also includes school health services, social work services in schools, and parent counseling and training.	34 C.F.R. § 300.16(a)
Physical Therapy	Services provided by a qualified physical therapist.	34 C.F.R. § 300.16(a)(7)
Occupational Therapy	Includes–(i) improving, developing or restoring functions impaired or lost through illness, injury, or deprivation; (ii) improving ability to perform tasks for independent functioning when functions are impaired or lost; and (iii) preventing, through early intervention, initial or further impairment or loss of function.	34 C.F.R. § 300.16(a)(5)
Least Restrictive Environment	(1) To the maximum extent appropriate, children with disabilities, including children in public or private institutions or other care facilities, are educated with children who are nondisabled; and (2) that special classes, separate schooling or other removal of children	34 C.F.R. § 300.550(b)

Term	Definition	Citation–Code of Federal Regulations
	with disabilities from regular classes occurs only when the nature or severity of the disability is such that education in the regular classroom with the use of supplementary aids and services cannot be achieved satisfactorily.	
Assistive Technology	Each public agency shall ensure that assistive technology devices or assistive technology services, or both, as those terms are defined in §§ 300.5-300.6, are made available to a child with a disability if required as a part of the child's–(a) Special education under § 300.17; (b) Related services under § 300.16; or (c) Supplementary aids and services under § 300.550(b)(2).	34 C.F.R. § 300.308
Assistive Technology Device	Any item, piece of equipment, or product system, whether acquired commercially off the shelf, modified, or customized, that is used to increase, maintain, or improve the functional capabilities of children with disabilities.	34 C.F.R. § 300.5
Assistive Technology Service	Any service that directly assists a child with a disability in the selection, acquisition, or use of an assistive technology device. The term includes–(a) The evaluation of the needs of a child with a disability, including a functional evaluation of the child in the child's customary environment; (b) Purchasing, leasing, or otherwise providing for the acquisition of assistive technology devices by children with disabilities; (c) Selecting, designing, fitting, customizing, adapting, applying, retaining, repairing, or replacing assistive technology devices; (d) Coordinating and using other therapies, interventions, or services with assistive technology devices, such as those associated with existing education and	34 C.F.R. § 300.6

TABLE 1 (continued)

Term	Definition	Citation – Code of Federal Regulations
	rehabilitation plans and programs; (e) Training or technical assistance for a child with a disability or, if appropriate, that child's family; and (f) Training or technical assistance for professionals (including individuals providing education or rehabilitation services), employers, or other individuals who provide services to, employ, or are otherwise substantially involved in the major life functions of children with disabilities.	
Individualized Education Program	A written statement for a child with a disability that is developed and implemented in accordance with §§ 300.341-300.350.	34 C.F.R. § 300.340
Content of Individualized Education Program	The IEP for each child must include–(1) A statement of the child's present levels of educational performance; (2) A statement of annual goals, including short-term instructional objectives; (3) A statement of the specific special education and related services to be provided to the child and the extent that the child will be able to participate in regular educational programs; (4) The projected dates for initiation of services and the anticipated duration of the services; and (5) Appropriate objective criteria and evaluation procedures and schedules for determining, on at least an annual basis, whether the short-term instructional objectives are being achieved.	34 C.F.R. § 300.346

TABLE 2. Definitions from the Individuals with Disabilities Education Act (IDEA)–Part H (Infants and Toddlers with Disabilities)

Term	Definition	Citation–Code of Federal Regulations
Early Intervention Program	The total effort in a state that is directed at meeting the needs of children eligible under this part and their families.	34 C.F.R. § 303.11
Physical Therapy	Includes services to address the promotion of sensorimotor function through enhancement of musculoskeletal status, neurobehavioral organization, perceptual and motor development, cardiopulmonary status, and effective environmental adaptation.*	34 C.F.R. § 303.12(d)(9)
Occupational Therapy	Includes services to address the functional needs of a child related to adaptive development, adaptive behavior and play, and sensory, motor, and postural development. These services are designed to improve the child's functional ability to perform tasks in home, school, and community settings.**	34 C.F.R. § 303.12(d)(8)
Natural Environments	(1) To the maximum extent appropriate to the needs of the child, early intervention services must be provided in natural environments, including the home and community settings in which children without disabilities participate; (2) Settings that are natural or normal for the child's age peers who have no disability.	34 C.F.R. § 303.12(b)
Individualized Family Service Plan	A written plan for providing early intervention services to a child eligible under this part and the child's family.	34 C.F.R. § 303.340(b)
Content of an IFSP	The IFSP must include the following: (a) Information about the child's status; (b) Family information; (c) Outcomes; (d) Early intervention services; (e) Other services; (f) Dates; (g) Service coordinator; and (h) Transition from Part H services.***	34 C.F.R. § 303.344

*Additional information pertaining to the delivery of physical therapy services for infants and toddlers with disabilities can be found in 34 C.F.R. § 303.12(d)(9).

**Additional information pertaining to the delivery of occupational therapy services for infants and toddlers with disabilities can be found in 34 C.F.R. § 303.12(d)(8).

***Additional information pertaining to the content of IFSP for infants and toddlers with disabilities can be found in 34 C.F.R. § 303.344.

FIGURE 3. Due Process Procedure and Judicial Interpretation

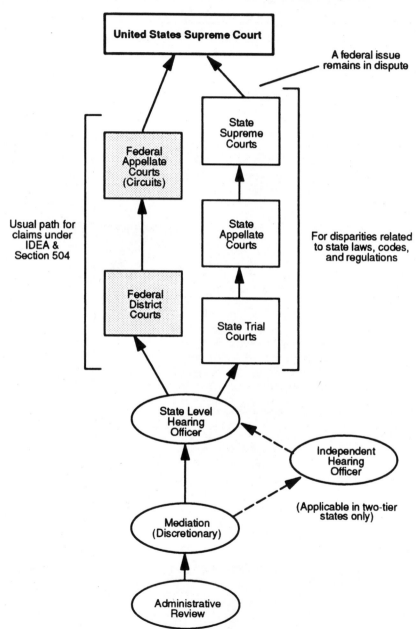

state levels, either party may eventually seek a decision through the federal or state judicial systems.

Essentially, two separate and distinct judicial paths exist to obtain a remedy under the laws that provide special education and related services: state courts and federal courts. Claims that contain issues pertaining exclusively to state laws, codes, and regulations are tried in the state court system with the state supreme court acting as the final arbitrator at this level. Disparities that involve federal statutes and regulations enter the federal judicial system, and the United States Supreme Court provides the final point of appeal for federal cases. Occasionally, a state case will be appealed to the Supreme Court when all state issues are resolved and a federal issue remains in dispute.

Eligibility for Special Education Services

IDEA provides a free, appropriate public education (FAPE), including special education and related services, to all eligible children with disabilities regardless of the nature and severity of the disability.[12] Children with disabilities are defined as those having a disability that adversely affects educational performance and who otherwise meet the existing definitions for one of the 13 disability categories (autism, deaf-blindness, deafness, hearing impairment, mental retardation, multiple disabilities, orthopedic impairment, other health impairment, serious emotional disturbance, specific learning disability, speech or language impairment, traumatic brain injury, and visual impairment) included in the federal statute.[13] Qualifying children with disabilities are eligible to receive all related services, including physical therapy and occupational therapy, that have been determined to be necessary to assist them to benefit from special education.

In addition to the 13 disability categories listed above, Part B allows for the use of the categorical label "developmental delay" with children ages 3 through 5 at the discretion of each state.[14] Therefore, each state is responsible for developing, approving, and providing their own definition and criteria for the developmental delay label.

Individualized Education Program

The Individualized Education Program (IEP), a written document that reflects a cooperative agreement between the school district and parent, is established at an IEP meeting and should contain input from related service professionals who provide assessment, intervention, or both, to a child with disabilities. The evaluation of a child must be performed by a multidisciplinary team and must include a teacher or other specialist with knowledge in the area of each suspected disability.[15] As a result, the assessment of a child with a suspected motor disability would be likely to include a physical therapist or occupational therapist (or both) as the specialist with knowledge in motor abilities. The inclusion or exclusion of therapy services on the IEP of a child with motor disabilities cannot be assumed by other members of the IEP team who are not otherwise qualified to assess motor abilities and the need for intervention in this area. In one such situation, a school district was found to be in violation for not providing a FAPE when the school principal made a unilateral decision to exclude physical therapy services from the IEP of a child with a physical impairment.[16] In addition, when the need for therapy services has been identified by a specialist with knowledge in the area of the suspected disability, the delivery of the appropriate service(s) becomes the obligation of the school district in order to comply with IDEA,[17] regardless of whether the services are provided by district employees or through a contractual arrangement between the district and an outside agency. Prior history within a school district of not providing a particular related service (e.g., physical therapy, occupational therapy, orientation and mobility training, or sign language interpretation) does not alter the requirement to provide the service should an IEP team determine its necessity as part of a child's special education program.

Related service personnel are not required to attend IEP meetings even when such services have been determined to be necessary to provide a FAPE to a child with disabilities. When the qualified provider of a related service is unable to attend the IEP meeting, however, a written recommendation that includes the nature (e.g., direct, indirect, or consultative), frequency (e.g., number of times per week or month), and amount of service (e.g., number of minutes) to be provided to the child should be developed and forwarded to the IEP team prior to the meeting.[18] The practice of providing a written report in lieu of attending and directly participating in an IEP meeting is not advisable, however, because it requires the therapist, in absentia, to provide recommendations on service delivery without the benefit of participating in the team meeting about the child's educational program. Additionally, this practice requires other IEP team members to integrate the information and rationale provided by an absent member of the team.

The information provided by a therapist either prior to, or at, an IEP meeting must include the child's present level of performance and any other factors that will assist the team in developing realistic annual goals and short-term objectives. This process of developing goals and objectives after assessing the child's function is intended to create a direct link between the child's present level of function and the intervention that will assist the child in accomplishing positive post-school outcomes as a result of the specially designed instructional program. The IEP must be reviewed annually,[19] although it may be reviewed and altered more frequently should the need arise. Any member of the IEP team, including a therapist, may initiate the process to reconvene the IEP team for a meeting to modify goals and objectives, request a change of placement, or otherwise alter the nature or delivery of the child's program.[20]

Providing Related Services

The federal definition of related services in IDEA differentiates between those services that are necessary for a child to receive educational benefit and those services that are not a fundamental part of the child's program by including the phrase "to assist a child with disabilities to benefit from special education" in the definition.[5] Special education is defined as "specially designed instruction, at no cost to the parents, to meet the unique needs of a child with a disability."[21] Specially designed instruction for a child with a disability may, in fact, be physical therapy or occupational therapy to meet the child's unique needs. When physical and/or occupational therapy are the specially designed instruction, and state regulations permit, these services may be provided as a child's special education program rather than as a related service to another stand-alone component of the child's specially designed instructional program.[22] For example, Ohio's *Rules for the Education of Handicapped Children*[23] defines special education as a term that "includes speech and language services or any other related service, if the services consist of specially designed instruction, at no cost to the parent, to meet the unique needs of a handicapped child . . ." (p. 12). Accordingly, these services are then considered "special education" rather than a "related service" when provided as the child's specially designed instructional program. Although New Mexico[24] shares a similar definition to that provided in Ohio, Rhode Island[25] and Oklahoma permit only speech-language pathology to stand alone as a child's special education program. An examination of *Policies and Procedures for Special Education in Oklahoma*[26] indicates that no other related services are included in the definition of special education.

Federal statutes do not require special education programs to provide a level of service or meet a standard that maximizes educational opportunities for children with disabilities. In fact, IDEA only requires that children receive "some educational benefit" from their special education program. This judicial interpretation of congressional intent in making public education available to all children was summarized during one of the landmark cases in special education, *Board of Educ. of the Hendrick Hudson Cent. Sch. Dist. v. Rowley.*[27] The federal law provides a "basic floor of opportunity"[28] and does not require maximizing a child's potential except when state statutes require that this higher standard be met. The *Rowley* case involved a young girl with a hearing impairment whose parents requested the provision of a sign language interpreter as a related service to support their daughter's specially designed instructional program. Amy Rowley exhibited satisfactory academic progress in school without the assistance of an interpreter. It was, therefore, presumed that she was deriving some educational benefit. The Court's decision[28] clearly indicated that Amy was not entitled to additional related services when those services were not necessary to provide her with a basic floor of opportunity to support educational achievement.

Similar reasoning may be applied to other related services. When physical and/or occupational therapy services are necessary components of an educational program that provides a child with a basic floor of opportunity-access to an equal opportunity which would not otherwise exist without these therapy services-and not merely maximization of a child's potential, these therapy services are considered to be necessary for a FAPE and provided at no cost to parents. A child, such as Douglas, might receive occupational therapy to improve upper extremity function necessary to achieve his educational goals. Conversely, a child with mild hemiplegia that does not adversely affect educational performance and functional use of both arms probably will not be eligible for occupational therapy provided by the school district at no cost to parents. Eligibility for services cannot be based on parental desire for additional therapy to refine motor control of the nondominant extremity when the goal is not essentially linked to educational benefit.

Delivery of Special Education and Related Services

Special education is not a place; it is the specially designed instruction that reflects the program and services identified by the IEP team and committed by the local school district that will be provided to a child with disabilities. Figure 4 graphically describes the appropriate pathway for determining a child's needs prior to developing a program. The first step involves an appropriate evaluation by a multidisciplinary team that includes testing in the child's native language and assessment in all areas related to the suspected disability.[15] Following an evaluation, the IEP team will develop an appropriate program based on long-term goals and short-term objectives generated after considering the child's current level of

FIGURE 4. Pathway to Providing Special Education and Related Services

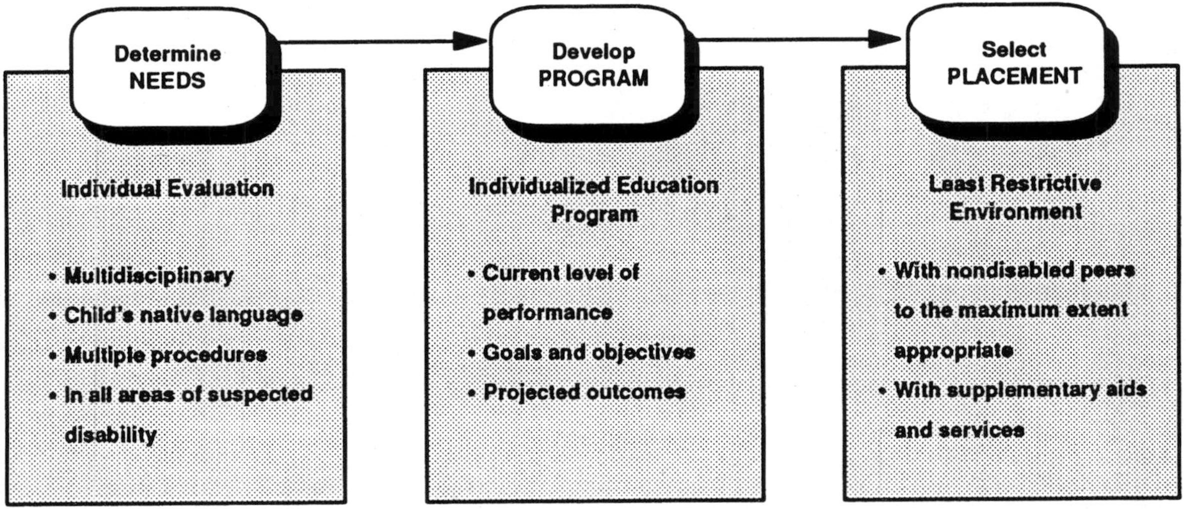

Determine NEEDS

Individual Evaluation

- Multidisciplinary
- Child's native language
- Multiple procedures
- In all areas of suspected disability

Develop PROGRAM

Individualized Education Program

- Current level of performance
- Goals and objectives
- Projected outcomes

Select PLACEMENT

Least Restrictive Environment

- With nondisabled peers to the maximum extent appropriate
- With supplementary aids and services

function and projected future outcomes. A decision pertaining to placement should be made only when the two prior steps in the sequence have been completed.

As part of the IEP process, decisions are also made regarding the frequency and nature of all necessary related services. The school district commits its financial and personnel resources to the delivery of these services through the IEP process. The provision of related services, like specially designed instruction, must be determined based on individual need. Children cannot be provided a predetermined level of service that has been based on a categorical or disability label.[29] For example, just as a 180-day school year is not appropriate for all children with disabilities,[30,31,32,33,34] neither should all children with multiple disabilities automatically receive individualized direct (one-to-one) occupational therapy for 30 minutes per week or therapy one time per month in a small group. Nor should children with a particular diagnosis or who are a particular age automatically receive consultative physical therapy services. Each child's program must be designed around the unique need of the individual child in order to deliver a FAPE.

While one child may require direct and frequent intervention, another child's needs might be adequately served through therapy services delivered in a consultative model in the classroom.[35,36] School districts may be in violation of not delivering a FAPE when therapy services are included on a child's IEP but are not provided. In one situation, a one-month delay in initiating occupational therapy was cause for the school district to be found in violation by the Office of Civil Rights (OCR).[37] In a related case, a delay in initiating occupational therapy cost a school district over $14,000 in reimbursement for therapy services parents obtained outside the educational setting and for legal fees for both the school district and the parents (as the prevailing party).[38] A school district was also found to be responsible for financial reimbursement to parents for the expenses they incurred when physical therapy for their child with multiple disabilities was reduced from direct intervention 3 times per week to intervention only 2 times per week.[39] The amount of service (i.e., 3 times per week), which had been determined to be necessary by the IEP team, was reduced by the district administration for the sake of administrative expediency and not because the child's needs had changed.

There have been, and continue to be, situations in which parents request specific therapy services from the school district for their child. The requested services may be beyond: (a) the amount of service able to be provided in school; (b) the expertise of the therapists employed or contracted by the school district; or (c) the essential components of the child's educational program as determined by the other members of the IEP team. Frequently, the requests for these services mirror interventions that are more typically delivered by a therapist in a setting outside the school environment (e.g., in a hospital or outpatient clinic). The use of a particular treatment may be espoused by a therapist in a clinical setting and suggested by the parents as the treatment "of choice" during an IEP meeting. On occasion, the courts have recognized and accepted the need for providing such services outside the educational environment when the necessary service is appropriate for the child, as determined by the IEP team, and when it cannot be provided by the school district.[40] However, this is not the case with many of the requests for alternative models of therapeutic intervention. A recent hearing officer's decision held that a student was not entitled to horseback riding as a therapeutic modality at school district expense when the same goals and objectives offered by the horseback riding program could be addressed by a more traditional physical therapy program delivered in the school environment by the school-based therapist.[41] Decisions regarding the need for therapy services, as well as the nature and frequency of the intervention, are made as part of the child's IEP.

Least Restrictive Environment

A child's disability label or the type of service required by the child does not determine the child's placement (refer to Figure 4). Congress has recognized the need to educate all children in the least restrictive environment based on a continuum of placements. Education in the least restrictive environment requires that children with disabilities be educated in the regular classroom with nondisabled peers to the maximum extent appropriate and may include the use of supplemental aids and services to achieve this goal.[42] In addition, children with disabilities are to attend the closest accessible school unless their IEP requires otherwise.[43] Therefore, a child who has an orthopedic impairment requiring the use of a walker for ambulation, the services of a tutor for one hour per day, bus transportation for the 3/4 mile trip from home to school, and physical therapy for 30 minutes per week should only be removed from the closest accessible school when the IEP cannot be delivered in that environment. The burden of proof rests with the school district to either deliver the IEP in the closest accessible school or prove why this placement would not be appropriate prior to sending the child to another building in the district or to an out-of-district site. Furthermore, related services, as part of the special education program, should be delivered in the least restrictive environment unless the IEP goals, and hence the intervention, require otherwise.

A child with cerebral palsy who receives occupational therapy to work on dressing, feeding, and visual-motor skills should be able to receive these services in the home school (i.e., closest accessible school the child would attend if nondisabled) unless other needs prevent the placement. The need for occupational therapy or physical therapy does not, in and of itself, justify placement at another school building. Therapists must be concerned with providing services in the least restrictive environment and with supporting a child's special education program and learning environment.

Transition

As related service providers, therapists may need to be involved with several clearly identified phases of transition for children with disabilities. Transition of children from IDEA Part H to Part B must be completed by the child's third birthday[44] for those children who are eligible for preschool programs under Part B. The transition process is designed to ensure the uninterrupted provision of services from one program or agency to another. Related service providers may be essential in facilitating a smooth transition for a child who is receiving early intervention services under Part H in a home-based program and who will begin attending a center-based program for three-year-olds under Part B. Consider the example of a 32 month old child who is medically fragile and developmentally delayed and for whom the vulnerability to frequent childhood illnesses justifies the need for a home-based early intervention program. As the child's third birthday approaches and the child becomes more medically stable, a move into a center-based program is appropriate. During this transitional period, therapists may: (a) prepare center staff to meet the child's needs, including accommodations related to mobility, feeding, toileting, positioning, etc.; (b) evaluate the building, classroom, and play areas for accessibility and provide suggestions for necessary changes; and (c) communicate with therapists who provide services at the center to discuss the child's progress, Part H goals, and level of function.

In addition, related service providers may be involved with the transition of students from school to post-school activities for students with disabilities age 16 and older who are eligible for special education and related services under IDEA. Transition planning may begin for students at a younger age when appropriate[45] and provides a structure for the team to identify needed services and responsible agencies prior to graduation from high school or the student's twenty-first birthday, whichever comes first. Clearly, not all recipients of special education under IDEA, Part B, will need transition services, but the option must be available. The decision to forego developing a specific transition plan must be made on an individual basis by the IEP team. The absence of a statement of needed transition services on the IEP of a student age 16 or older should be justified by documenting that the team gave individual consideration to the child's current level of performance and transition-related needs prior to deciding that a transition plan was not necessary.

Physical therapy and occupational therapy services may be part of the transition process to address some of the following: mobility in community environments, access and use of public transportation, job skills and performance, acquisition of necessary technology and equipment, and access to community agencies, programs, and services for adults. The mandate to include a statement of needed transition services and the provision of assistive technology devices and services has been included in IDEA since the 1990 Amendments.

Assistive Technology Services

Prior to being included within IDEA statutory and regulatory provisions, assistive technology devices and services were recognized for the important role they can play in fostering quality of life and independence for individuals with disabilities. The Technology-Related Assistance for Individuals with Disabilities Act (commonly known as the Tech Act)[46] was originally passed in 1988 and reauthorized in 1993. IDEA adopted its basic terminology and concepts in providing assistive technology to children with disabilities from the Tech Act[47] and implemented the provision as part of the educational program for children who require such assistance as part of a FAPE. Assistive technology devices and services are available to a child with a disability if required as part of the child's special education program, as a related service to assist a child to benefit from their special education program, or as supplementary aids and services in the regular classroom.[48] The obligation of acquiring (not necessarily purchasing) assistive technology devices and providing assistive technology services remains with the school district or Local Education Agency (LEA) when the IEP team has determined that assistive technology is necessary for the delivery of a FAPE.

Assistive technology service[49] is the process of assisting a child with disabilities in the selection, acquisition, or use of an assistive technology device (refer to Table 1). This may include evaluation of the child's needs related to assistive technology, as well as fitting and adapting an existing or newly purchased device, and providing training or technical assistance for people who may be involved with the major life functions of a child who uses an assistive technology device.[49] These services are likely to be performed primarily by related service personnel, including physical therapists and occupational therapists, particularly for children with moderate and severe disabilities. Speech-language pathologists are also frequently involved in providing assistive technology services related to the evaluation, acquisition, and use of augmentative communication devices. Rainforth, York, and Macdonald[50] have addressed the benefits of transdisciplinary evaluation and intervention for children with severe disabilities. The transdisciplinary approach involving a variety of professionals from various disciplines can be particularly effective for the evaluation, acquisition, and use of assistive technology devices in schools.

Alternative Funding Sources

It is not surprising that many school districts have looked to alternative funding sources to supplement the limited financial contribution provided by the federal government and state legislatures for the delivery of special education and related services to children with disabilities under IDEA. In fact, IDEA speaks to the importance of developing and implementing interagency agreements between the State Education Agency (SEA) and other state and local agencies that may be involved with providing or paying for a FAPE.[51] Many school districts are accessing Medicaid and private insurance funds as sources of financial reimbursement for the delivery of related services provided to children with disabilities as part of a FAPE.[52,53] In 1992, the U.S. Department of Health and Human Services (HHS), in cooperation with the Health Care Financing Administration (HCFA) and the Office of Special Education and Rehabilitative Services (OSERS), issued a policy clarification document[54] to provide state and local education agencies with the information necessary to proceed with third party reimbursement from Medicaid for appropriate related services to eligible children with IEPs.

As the process of accessing alternative funding sources by school districts and special education or therapy cooperatives becomes more common, numerous obstacles have emerged. These include: (a) extensive documentation required of therapists that can be tedious, time consuming, and hence costly as a use of therapists' billable hours; and (b) requirements set forth by Medicaid and private insurance companies that may preclude the delivery of therapy services consistent with the child's special education program as determined by the IEP team. For example, alternative funding sources may not be receptive to providing reimbursement for the delivery of services to multiple children who are seen simultaneously in a small group or the provision of services using a consultative service delivery model.

Interested readers may want to pursue the identified references for further information.

SECTION 504 OF THE REHABILITATION ACT OF 1973

Children who qualify as individuals with disabilities under Section 504 of the Rehabilitation Act of 1973[3] may be entitled to reasonable accommodations in the educational program by nature of the protection guaranteed them as a protected class under basic civil rights law (refer to Figure 2). Under Section 504, an individual with disabilities (a) has a physical or mental impairment that substantially limits one or more major life activities; (b) has a record of having a physical or mental impairment that substantially limits one or more major life activities; or (c) is not impaired but is regarded as having such an impairment.[55] Children who meet the definition of having a disability under Section 504,[56] but who would not otherwise be eligible for special education and related services under IDEA because the disability does not adversely affect educational performance, form the class for which reasonable accommodations may be necessary under Section 504. Children with disabilities are not eligible for specialized instruction and related services under IDEA unless the nature of the disability is such that it has an adverse affect on educational performance (e.g., child's increasing weakness results in decreasing educational performance). Section 504 provides another avenue for accommodation for some children with disabilities. An example of the need for physical therapy as a reasonable accommodation under Section 504 might involve consultation by a therapist with a classroom teacher and/or building administrator regarding a safe and efficient plan for evacuation of a child who has a mobility impairment, but does not require special education, from the school building in an emergency situation. Additional criteria to determine eligibility of children for protection under Section 504 require that the child (a) be of an age during which all children without disabilities would receive such services, (b) be of an age during which the state provides a FAPE, or (c) be of an age during which it is mandatory to provide such services to individuals with disabilities.[57] Only the second and third criteria have a relevant connection to the delivery of physical therapy and occupational therapy in schools.

As a result, physical therapy or occupational therapy, particularly consultative services for a child with a mild disability, would be considered to be a reasonable accommodation under Section 504. Another example may be helpful: A young girl with myelomeningocele successfully attends her neighborhood elementary school. She performs at grade level without any special services or accommodations. She ambulates independently using Lofstrand crutches around the elementary school building and to all special subjects and extracurricular activities. The elementary school building is all on ground level with only a single step to enter the front door of the building. Beginning with the next academic year, she will attend middle school at an older three-story building. Her physical needs are consistently monitored by her physician and the therapists associated with the myelomeningocele clinic she attends every 6 months. Recognizing the upcoming change in buildings and a more challenging terrain, the girl's parents have asked the school district for a physical therapy consultation during the spring semester of the current academic year to assess their daughter's ability to move independently about the middle school building. This consultation would allow school district administrators to make any adaptations in room assignments or in the girl's schedule prior to the start of the next school year. The physical therapy consultation could be provided as part of a 504 Plan that may resemble an IEP, but which is developed and implemented under Section 504[58] to meet the needs of a child with a disability that does not adversely affect educational performance. An IEP is not necessary as this child does not require special education or related services as part of FAPE under IDEA.

Although many simple accommodations (e.g., rest time during the school day, availability of a private restroom facility for catheterization, consultative services by related service providers) can be made under Section 504, school districts may be reluctant to offer such provisions without formally identifying and labeling students with disabilities. Section 504 requires compliance by federal recipients, but the statute does not provide financial reimbursement or incentives for accommodative services which are required to comply with the law. Identification of students under IDEA following an evaluation and subsequent development of an IEP provides for minimal reimbursement to school districts from federal and state resources. Failure to comply with Section 504 can only result in loss of federal funds and federal contracts. The Office of Civil Rights (OCR) is the federal agency responsible for investigating and issuing formal citations for violations that have resulted in limiting equal opportunities for individuals with disabilities.

THE AMERICANS WITH DISABILITIES ACT

A more recent, and more global, protection of civil rights for individuals with disabilities is contained in the Americans with Disabilities Act, which was passed and signed into law in 1990.[4] The definition of an individual with disabilities from Section 504 is mirrored in the ADA,[59] however, the protection is broadened by the scope of the legislation to encompass both public and private entities. The greatest implications for related service providers working with children in the educational environment are two-fold: (1) protection is available to any therapist who meets the definition of an individual with a disability in obtaining and maintaining employment by requesting reasonable accommodations, and (2) therapists who are involved with vocational training and postsecondary transition should understand the level of compliance required by businesses and postsecondary educational institutions in the community. Reasonable accommodations[60] (those modifications or adjustments that do not cause undue hardship and do not alter the fundamental nature of the position or business) are required by agencies and businesses in the hiring of qualified persons with disabilities,[61] although smaller businesses (those with less than fifteen employees) are exempt from providing any accommodations under the ADA.[62] The definitions and specific criteria for "reasonable accommodation"[61] and "undue hardship"[63] continue to be interpreted through judicial decisions and legislative actions. The impact of the ADA on therapy services in educational environments has been minimal to date.

CONCLUSION

Understanding the laws that shape the delivery of therapy services in schools is one of the essential components leading to best practice by physical therapists and occupational therapists employed in educational environments. Most of the children who receive therapy in educational environments have disabilities that adversely affect their educational performance; hence, their rights and the rights of their parents are protected under IDEA. When a child is eligible under IDEA, therapy services will be part of a specially designed instructional program that has been developed, approved, and implemented by an IEP team. As related services, physical therapy and occupational therapy services are linked to the child's educational program and may also be necessary to assist the child to meet the environmental demands of the educational environment in conjunction with providing the child a FAPE. Special education and related services are provided at no cost to parents, and each child's program should be designed to meet individual needs. As a result, the frequency and nature of school-based therapy services may vary widely from one child to another.

Children with disabilities may also receive therapy as a reasonable accommodation in the educational environment even when a disability has not been shown to adversely affect educational performance. Though this situation is much less common, therapists should be aware of and understand the implications for service delivery presented by Section 504 of the Rehabilitation Act and the Americans with Disabilities Act. These civil rights statutes afford children and adults with disabilities equal opportunity (not necessarily identical results or levels of achievement) and may include the provision of therapy services as a means of creating or maintaining such opportunity.

Although this paper has focused almost exclusively on federal laws, therapists should also be familiar with statutes, regulations, and policies within the state of licensure and where services are being delivered to insure that all criteria for service delivery are adequately met.

REFERENCES

1. *Individuals with Disabilities Education Act of 1990*, 20 USC §1400-1485.

2. Assistance to States for the Education of Children with Disabilities Program and Preschool Grants for Children with Disabilities; Final Rule (34 CFR Parts 300 and 301). *Federal Register* 1992; 57 (Sept 29): 44794-44852.

3. *Section 504 of the Rehabilitation Act of 1973*, 29 USC §794.

4. *Americans with Disabilities Act of 1990*, 42 USC §12101.

5. 34 CFR §300.16 (a).

6. 34 CFR §§300.16 (a)(5), 300.16 (a)(7).

7. 34 CFR §300.12 (d)(9).

8. 34 CFR §303.1.

9. 34 CFR §303.16 (b).

10. *The Education of All Handicapped Children Act*, Amendments of 1986, Public Law 99-457.

11. 34 CFR § 303.12.

12. *Individuals with Disabilities Education Act of 1990*, 20 USC §1412 (2)(C).

13. *Individuals with Disabilities Education Act of 1990*, 20 USC §1401 (1)(A).

14. 34 CFR §300.7 (a)(2).

15. 34 CFR § 300.532.

16. *Pittsburgh Bd. of Ed. v. Commonwealth, Dept. of Educ.*, 581 A.2d 681 (Pa. Commw. Ct. 1990).

17. Assistance to States for the Education of Children with Disabilities Program and Preschool Grants for Children with Disabilities; Final Rule (34 CFR Parts 300 and 301). *Federal Register* 1992; 57 (Sept 29): 44838, Appendix C, Number 45.

18. Assistance to States for the Education of Children with Disabilities Program and Preschool Grants for Children with Disabilities; Final Rule (34 CFR Parts 300 and 301). *Federal Register.* 1992; 57 (Sept 29): 44836, Appendix C, Number 23.

19. *Individuals with Disabilities Education Act of 1990*, 20 USC §1414 (a)(5).

20. 34 CFR §300.343 (11).

21. *Individuals with Disabilities Education Act of 1990*, 20 USC §1401 (a) (16).

22. 34 CFR §300.17 (a)(2).

23. Rules for the Education of Handicapped Children, 1982; Ohio Rev Code § 3301-51-01 (DDD).

24. Standards for Excellence in New Mexico Schools Compliance Manual, State Board of Education Regulations 90-2, New Mexico State Department of Education, 1992; Chapter 5 §5.12 (AC).

25. Regulations of the Board of Regents for Elementary and Secondary Education Governing the Special Education of Students with Disabilities, State of Rhode Island & Providence Plantations, 1992; §3.0, Note 1.

26. Policies and Procedures for Special Education in Oklahoma, Oklahoma State Department of Education, 1993; 3.

27. *Board of Educ. of the Hendrick Hudson Cent. Sch. Dist. v. Rowley*, 102 S. Ct. 3034, 3048 (1982).

28. *Board of Educ. of the Hendrick Hudson Cent. Sch. Dist. v. Rowley*, 458 US 176 (1982).

29. *Polk v. Susquehana Intermediate Unit 16*, 853 F.2d 171 (3d Cir. 1988).

30. Rapport MJ, Thomas SB: Extended school year: Legal issues and implications. *Journal of The Association for Persons with Severe Handicaps.* 1993;18: 16-27.

31. *Armstrong v. Kline*, 476 F. Supp. 583 (E.D. Pa. 1979), *aff'd sub nom., Battle v. Pennsylvania*, 629 F.2d 269 (3d Cir. 1980).

32. *Crawford v. Pittman*, 708 F.2d 1028 (5th Cir. 1983).

33. *Georgia Association of Retarded Citizens v. McDaniel*, 511 F. Supp. 1263 (N.D. Ga. 1981), *aff'd*, 716 F.2d 1565 (11th Cir. 1983).

34. *Yaris v. Special School District of St. Louis County*, 545 (E.D. Mo. 1983), *aff'd*, 728 F.2d 1055 (8th Cir. 1984).

35. *In re: Beth Ann P.*, 16 EHLR 60 (SEA Pa. 1989).

36. *Summers Cty. (WV) Sch.*, 20 IDELR 1362 (OCR 1993).

37. *Brockton (MA) Pub. Sch.*, 20 IDELR 914 (OCR 1993).

38. *Rapid City Sch. Dist. 51/4 v. Vahle*, 733 F.2d 476 (8th Cir. 1990).

39. *In re A Child with Disabilities*, 21 IDELR 594 (SEA Ct. 1994).

40. *Das v. McHenry Sch. Dist. No. 15*, 20 IDELR 979 (N.D. Ill. 1994).

41. *East Windsor Bd. of Ed.*, 20 IDELR 1478 (SEA Ct. 1994).

42. *Individuals with Disabilities Education Act of 1990*, 20 USC §1412 (5)(B).

43. 34 CFR §300.552.

44. 34 CFR §303.148 (b)(2).

45. 34 CFR §300.346 (b)(1).

46. *Technology-Related Assistance for Individuals with Disabilities Act of 1988*, 29 USC § 2201.

47. 34 CFR §300.6, Note; *Federal Register* 1992;57 (Sept 29):44801.

48. 34 CFR §300.308.

49. 34 CFR §300.6.

50. Rainforth B, York J, Macdonald C: *Collaborative Teams for Students with Severe Disabilities: Integrating Therapy and Educational Services.* Baltimore, MD: Paul H. Brookes Publishing Co.; 1992.

51. *Individuals with Disabilities Education Act of 1990,* 20 USC §1413 (1) (13).

52. Kreb R: *Third Party Payment for Funding Special Education and Related Services.* Horsham, PA: LRP Publications; 1991.

53. Rogers J: *Third Party Billing for Special Education: Panacea or Mirage?* Cambridge, MA: Brookline Books; 1993.

54. HHS Policy Clarification, 18 IDELR 558 (HHS 1992).

55. 34 CFR, §104.3 (j)(1).

56. 34 CFR, §104.3 (j)(2).

57. 34 CFR, §104.3 (k)(2).

58. Zirkel PA: *Section 504 and the Schools.* Horsham, PA: LRP Publications; 1993: Appendix 5:12.

59. 29 CFR §1630.2(g).

60. 29 CFR §1630.2(o).

61. 29 CFR §1630.2(m).

62. 29 CFR §1630.2(e).

63. 29 CFR §1630.2(n).

Pediatric Therapy in the 1990s: The Demise of the Educational versus Medical Dichotomy

Irene R. McEwen

M'Lisa L. Shelden

SUMMARY. Since Public Law 94-142 was enacted in 1975, occupational therapists, physical therapists, parents, school administrators, physicians, and others have questioned and debated the difference between "medical therapy" and "educational therapy." This article proposes that changes in pediatric therapy in the 1990s have made the issue moot. Contemporary models of motor development, motor control, and motor learning, combined with an emphasis on functional outcomes and family-centered services, not only support current practices in special education, but pertain to children receiving therapy services in any setting. *[Article copies available from The Haworth Document Delivery Service: 1-800-342-9678.]*

Discussions about occupational therapy and physical therapy in educational environments usually turn to an attempt to define the differences

---

Irene R. McEwen, PhD, PT, PCS, is Associate Professor, and M'Lisa L. Shelden, MEd, PT, PCS, is Adjunct Assistant Professor, Department of Physical Therapy, University of Oklahoma Health Sciences Center, P.O. Box 26901, Oklahoma City, OK 73190.

Partial support for preparation of this manuscript was provided by a Preparation of Related Services Personnel grant (#HO29F30020) from the U.S. Department of Education, Office of Special Education and Rehabilitative Services. The contents do not necessarily represent the policy of the agency, however, and no official endorsement should be inferred.

[Haworth co-indexing entry note]: "Pediatric Therapy in the 1990s: The Demise of the Educational versus Medical Dichotomy." McEwen, Irene R., and M'Lisa L. Shelden. Co-published simultaneously in *Physical & Occupational Therapy in Pediatrics* (The Haworth Press, Inc.) Vol. 15, No. 2, 1995, pp. 33-45; and: *Occupational and Physical Therapy in Educational Environments* (ed: Irene R. McEwen) The Haworth Press, Inc., 1995, pp. 33-45. Single or multiple copies of this article are available from The Haworth Document Delivery Service [1-800-342-9678, 9:00 a.m - 5:00 p.m. (EST)].

between "medical therapy" and "educational therapy." Although the dichotomy may have been real in the mid-1970s when most states implemented Public Law 94-142,[1] current views on therapy for school-age children and youth with disabilities have made the issue largely irrelevant. As will be discussed in this article, contemporary theories of motor development and motor control, with an emphasis on functional activities, support current models of service delivery in educational environments and also apply to children receiving therapy services in medical and clinical settings.

RECENT CHANGES IN PEDIATRIC THERAPY

Some of the greatest changes in pediatric therapy over the past 20 years have taken place in the 1990s. New understanding about how motor behaviors are controlled and learned, changes in attitudes about the role of families in service systems, and health care reform efforts have all contributed to three major shifts in pediatric therapy: (1) from neuromaturational and reflex-hierarchial models of assessment and intervention to systems models and motor learning principles; (2) from measuring within a neurodevelopmental framework to measuring within a disablement model that focuses on functional activities; and (3) from center-based and child-centered services to family-centered services in natural environments.[2]

Systems Models of Assessment and Intervention

Neuromaturational and reflex-hierarchial theories of motor development and motor control have had a major influence on pediatric therapeutic approaches since the 1960s, particularly for children with cerebral palsy and other developmental disabilities.[3,4] These theories are based primarily on the observed sequence of typical infant development and on the animal research of Sherrington, Magnus, and others who attempted to map the functions of various areas of the brain.[5] As a result, treatment principles based on the theories emphasize such concepts as the normal developmental sequence as a model for treatment, cephalocaudal and proximal to distal development, and use of sensory input to facilitate motor output. Inhibition of abnormal reflexes, tone, and patterns of movement is considered to be a prerequisite for improved motor function. Two of the most prominent neurofacilitation approaches in pediatric therapy, neurodevelopmental treatment and sensory integration therapy, were based on these principles.[5]

Recent research, however, has failed to support many of the neuromaturational and reflex-hierarchial foundations of the neurofacilitation approaches. The belief that motor development proceeds in cephalocaudal and proximal to distal directions, and from gross motor to fine motor skills, for example, has not been upheld.[6,7] Rather, motor control is now believed to develop relatively simultaneously and independently throughout the body. Development may appear to be directional, such as an infant gaining head control before trunk control, but factors other than cephalocaudal development have been shown to account for the timing of skill acquisition. Thelen[8] demonstrated, for example, that infants' kicking is actually more skilled than their arm movements, but they are able to use their arm movements earlier, such as for reach and grasp, because the balance, strength, and other components necessary to use legs for standing and walking develop at a later time.[9]

As research in the neurosciences has accumulated and merged with developments in cognitive psychology, motor learning, kinesiology, and biomechanics, older theories of motor behavior have been replaced with systems models.[3] Systems models view behavior, including motor behavior, as the end product of multiple internal and external components, or subsystems. Some of the subsystems identified by researchers as contributing to motor control include sensorimotor, cognitive, mechanical, and task variables.[10] In a developing child, each internal subsystem has its own nonlinear time table[3] and motor behaviors emerge when each subsystem has developed to the necessary extent. Subsystems involved in infant kicking, for example, may include nervous system maturation, arousal level, posture or position of the infant, and the task constraints.[9]

Another important concept of a systems approach is that motor behavior is organized to accomplish specific tasks within a particular context.[11,12] For this reason, useful motor behaviors are more likely to result from working on functional tasks than from working on movement patterns for movement's sake alone.[13] As Gordon said, it is easy to facilitate movement patterns; what is difficult is to get people to use the pattern during some functional activity.[14] It is unlikely, for example, that movement organized to maintain balance while sitting on a ball will be helpful in maintaining balance while sitting on a chair to work at a computer or standing in line at a drinking fountain. Sitting on a ball, sitting on a chair, and standing in line are different tasks and movement is uniquely organized to accomplish each of them.[15]

Motor Learning and Teaching

Within a systems-based approach, motor learning principles provide direction for therapeutic intervention. Motor learning has been defined as processes associated with experience or practice that lead to relatively permanent changes in the capability for producing skilled action.[16] Motor behaviors that are retained for only a short period of time are not considered to be learned. Even though little of the motor learning research has been conducted with children with disabilities, studies of similar learning concepts have been reported in the education literature for many years.[17] As discussed below, transfer of behavior, organization of practice, and feedback are primary motor learning concepts that are being incorporated into therapeutic approaches.

Transfer of Behavior

Therapists and parents are often frustrated by children's inability to carry over motor behaviors exhibited during one therapy session to another therapy session or to function in everyday activities. Transfer of skills, in motor learning terms, or the concept of generalization in special education terms, refers to carry-over of behavior exhibited during one task or in one environment to a similar task in another environment.[16,18] Haring[19] defined generalization as the ability to respond appropriately in unrehearsed conditions, and described dimensions of generalization to include transfer of appropriate behaviors across persons, objects and materials, natural consequences, stimuli, settings, and time. A child who learns to walk between parallel bars, on a balance beam, or in a quiet therapy room, for example, must transfer or generalize to walking on a carpet at home or in a crowded hallway at school if walking is to be meaningful. Transfer must be actively programmed by the way in which practice is provided; it cannot be left to chance.[19,20]

Practice

Practice characteristics that have been found to enhance learning and transfer of skills are consistent with the systems perspective that motor behavior is goal-directed and organized within task-specific contexts. One of the most effective practice characteristics is to provide opportunities for practice in one or more environments in which the behavior will be used (or environments that are as similar to the real environment as possible) with natural consequences for the behavior. Practicing real stairs to get to lunch, for example, is more likely to be effective than practicing "stairs to nowhere" in the classroom or clinic. Practicing dressing in the locker room to go swimming is more likely to be effective than practicing dressing in a clinic or school therapy room.

Another important practice consideration is the organization of opportunities for practice. The motor learning literature uses the terms blocked practice and random practice, and the special education literature refers to essentially the same concepts as massed trials and distributed trials. Blocked practice and massed trials involve setting aside a certain period of time to practice a skill, such as using 10 minutes of twice weekly therapy sessions to practice standing from a sitting position. Random practice or distributed trials, in contrast, involve opportunities to practice a skill several times throughout a therapy session and as many times as possible throughout daily activities. Studies have shown that although blocked or massed practice may be beneficial for initial acquisition of a new skill, random or distributed practice is necessary for learning, recall, retention, and perfection of skill.[16,21] A child learning to drive a power wheelchair, for example, may benefit from blocked practice initially to learn how to move the chair, then practice throughout the day to promote retention of that skill and provide opportunities to further develop wheelchair driving skills. Another child who practices transferring from a wheelchair to a toilet each time she needs to go to the bathroom will learn to stand from sitting more readily and will learn to transfer more quickly than if practice is provided only during therapy sessions.

A sufficient number of opportunities to practice is critical if children are to develop motor skills. Think of the number of times a motorically gifted teenager might practice tennis serves, then think about the amount of practice that many children with disabilities receive. To provide enough opportunities, therapists must teach families and other service providers how to promote children's motor skills during activities that take place throughout the day. This is true regardless of whether the child receives services in school or in a clinical setting. Consultation and indirect models of service delivery (see Bundy, this volume) are often considered characteristic of school-based practice, but they are equally valuable for children receiving therapy in other settings.

Part-whole practice is another important motor learning concept.[22] Traditional neurofacilitation approaches often break motor tasks into component parts, such as working on trunk rotation on a bolster and squat to stand at an easel, then later attempting to put the pieces together. Sometimes the linking occurs within the same therapy session, often, though, the components are simply assumed to come together in the future. Research suggests that serial tasks that can be broken down into discrete motor elements, such as transferring from a wheelchair, may be learned effectively part by part (e.g., positioning the chair, locking the brakes, removing the armrest). Continuous tasks, such as walking, or discrete tasks, such as throwing, however, are best learned through practice of the whole task.[23]

Feedback

Feedback is another essential component of motor teaching and learning. With the neurofacilitation approaches, sensory input has traditionally been used to facilitate responses on an unconscious level. A child with cerebral palsy, for example, was supposed to become able to control head position automatically without use of cognitive processes. With motor learning approaches, intrinsic sensory feedback combined with visual, oral, and tactile extrinsic feedback are actively used by the child to solve motor problems.[5,24] Research suggests that judicious use of feedback is important, with continuous feedback perhaps beneficial for initial acquisition of a skill, but less frequent feedback important for learning and perfection of skill.

Overall, contemporary systems models of assessment and intervention, coupled with motor learning principles, support an emphasis on functional goals, intervention in natural environments, and organization of appropriate practice opportunities for children with disabilities. These concepts have long been a part of special education, but are now being recognized as fostering therapeutic outcomes as well as educational outcomes.

The Disablement Model

Disablement is a term that "reflects all of the diverse consequences that disease, injury, or congenital abnormalities may have on human functioning at many different levels."[25(p380)] For over 25 years, disablement schemes by Nagi[26] and the World Health Organization (WHO)[27] have influenced disability research in the United States,[25] but the application of these schemes to occupational therapy and physical therapy has been limited until recently. The *Pediatric Evaluation of Disability Inventory (PEDI)*[28] and the new book *Physical Therapy for Children*[29] are examples of the increasing influence and pediatric application of the disablement models over the past several years.

The five-component classification scheme by the National Center for Medical Rehabilitation Research (NCMRR),[30(p35)] which was adapted from the four-component Nagi[26] and the WHO[27] schemes, provides a useful framework for pediatric evaluation and intervention. The components or dimensions of the NCMRR model and their definitions are presented in Table 1, with an example of how each may be applied to a child with cerebral palsy.

A disablement scheme is helpful not only for determining the dimension(s) at which assessment and intervention should be targeted for the greatest impact, but it also clarifies how success of intervention must be measured. Intervention at the pathophysiology level is most often within the professional realm of physicians and biomedical researchers. Other than perhaps influencing brain structures of an infant through provision of critical experiences, occupational therapy and physical therapy begin their impact at the impairment component of the scheme.

Neurofacilitation approaches have traditionally focused assessment and intervention on primary impairment level phenomena, such as muscle tone, reflexes and automatic reactions, and responses to sensory stimuli.

TABLE 1. The National Center for Medical Rehabilitation Research (NCMRR)[30] Classification Schema Applied to a Child with Cerebral Palsy

---

Pathophysiology: Interruption of normal physiological and developmental processes or structures. *A child with cerebral palsy has brain damage or malformation.*

Impairment: Loss and/or abnormality of cognitive, emotional, physiological, or anatomical structure or function; includes secondary impairments not attributable to the initial pathophysiology. *As a result of pathophysiology, the child with cerebral palsy may have excess muscle contraction, and poor control of posture and balance, with a secondary impairment of range of motion limitations.*

Functional Limitations: Restriction or lack of ability to perform an action in the manner or range consistent with the purpose of an organ or organ system. *If a child's impairments are of sufficient magnitude, they will result in functional limitations, such as inability to reach, grasp, sit, or walk.*

Disability: Inability or limitation in performing tasks, activities, and roles to levels expected within physical and social contexts. Functional limitations may or may not lead to disability, or may lead to a disability under some conditions and not others. *A child with cerebral palsy who cannot walk may be able to fulfill expected roles related to mobility by using a wheelchair (not have a disability), but have a disability in other roles, such as self care.*

Societal Limitation: Restriction, attributable to social policy or barriers (structural or attitudinal), which limits fulfillment of roles or denies access to services and opportunities that are associated with full participation in society. *A child who uses a wheelchair but faces architectural barriers is limited by societal attitudes and actions.*

Little evidence exists to document that intervention at this level is effective for children with developmental disabilities, particularly beyond the first year or two of life. Rather, "it is time to let go of the concept of 'normalization' with respect to muscle tone, reflexes, and movement patterns, and work instead toward attainment of functional skills such as independence in mobility and communication."[31(p29)] Secondary impairments, such as deconditioning and contractures, which result from primary impairments and are usually not present in infants, need to be considered at any age.

Functional limitations, the next dimension of the model, are often documented by a child's failure to accomplish sitting, walking, dressing, or other age level skills listed on a developmental assessment. Most assessments and interventions conducted at this level are isolated from the context of functional activities that a child must perform to fulfill appropriate roles. Walking, for example, is usually evaluated apart from the role of moving from place to place within a natural environment. The *Gross Motor Function Measure*[32] is an example of a tool that examines functional limitations. Beyond early childhood it is probably not possible to modify functional limitations to a meaningful extent unless surgery, motivation, or some other event alters a critical subsystem of motor behavior. When intervention focuses on functional limitations, therapists often decide that an older child has reached a "plateau" when head control, sitting balance, or gait, for example, do not change and may recommend that therapy be discontinued. Refocusing on the disability or societal limitation dimensions often reveals important outcomes for children and youth of any age.

Disability assessment and intervention involve enabling children to assume age-appropriate roles to the fullest extent possible. In the top-down approach proposed by Campbell,[33] functional goals of intervention are identified first, then obstacles to accomplishing them are identified. These obstacles are often impairments or functional limitations, which can be directly targeted for intervention (if remediable) or bypassed through compensations, such as assistive technology or practicing a skill in spite of abnormal movement patterns. Therapists are often reluctant to pursue or even to permit use of compensations, but as Dunn proposes, "we need to embrace the approaches of promotion, prevention-intervention, and compensation as rigorously as we have embraced remediation in service provision."[34(p357)]

An example of assessment, intervention, and goals directed toward each dimension of the disablement scheme may help to clarify its application. Jim is a 6-year-old with cerebral palsy. Among other impairments, he has poor postural reactions which contribute to a functional limitation of being unable to sit independently. This functional limitation makes it impossible for Jim to assume a student's role with the rest of his class when they sit on the floor during opening circle, which is something he wants very much to do.

With a focus on the *impairment*, the therapist could identify Jim's poor postural reactions as a problem and attempt to improve them. A behavioral objective to reflect this effort might read:

> While sitting on a therapy ball, Jim will right himself when he is displaced laterally 20 degrees, 8 of 10 trials, by June, 199_.

Even if the objective is accomplished, it is unlikely that the learned motor behaviors will transfer or generalize to enable Jim to sit on the floor during circle time.

An objective focused on the *functional limitation* might be based on a failed item on a developmental test, such as:

> Jim will lean forward to get a toy without losing his balance or touching the floor on one of two trials by June, 199_.[35]

It is more likely that Jim will be able to sit on the floor during circle time if he can accomplish this objective, but it is not assured. By aiming directly at the *disability* with a top-down approach, the chances of Jim being able to sit on the floor and participate in circle time are much greater. If remediation is thought to be possible an objective could read:

> Jim will sit independently on his carpet square during opening circle and not fall over while he uses his communication board to answer questions for 5 consecutive school days by June, 199_.

By combining sitting with answering questions, the objective assures that sitting independently does not interfere with the part of his role that requires communication. If sitting demanded too much effort or attention, Jim might be able to sit, but be unable to do anything else at the same time. If remediation is not thought to be possible, a floor sitter or some other compensation could be provided that would bypass the motor obstacle and still permit him to accomplish the goal of sitting on the floor with the rest of the class.

The disablement model not only provides a framework for assessment and intervention for children with disabilities who receive therapy in clinical settings, but it is consistent with special education's focus on preparing students with disabilities to assume age-appropriate roles in their schools, communities, and homes. The disablement model is also consistent with the systems models and motor learning principles discussed previously, as well as with the shift from child-centered services to family-centered services.

Family-Centered Services

Health, education, and social service providers increasingly acknowledge the importance of involving "stakeholders" in the decisions and activities that affect them. A clear trend can be found in the general occupational therapy and physical therapy literature, for example, toward greater involvement of patients and their families in goal setting and intervention than in the past.[34,36] This trend is consistent with special education legislation, which has provided for expanded parental influence over the years, and with increased recognition by professionals that parents play a critical role in the development and well-being of their children.

Part H of the Individuals with Disabilities Education Act (IDEA) requires that early intervention services under its auspices be family-centered and provide families with the supports that they need to enhance their children's development.[37] This is in contrast to usual medical and special education (Part B) approaches, which focus on children's needs apart from the context of their families. Although special education has required parental involvement in placement and program decisions for more than 20 years, parents' input has often been ceremonial and limited to signing documents prepared by professionals. This is changing, though, as more children transition from family-centered early intervention programs to school and parents are demanding a continued voice in decisions that affect their children and families.

Family-centered services mean that families and children must be involved in identifying intervention goals that are meaningful to them and that intervention approaches clearly help to accomplish their desired outcomes. In pediatric therapy we have often assumed that our intervention will mysteriously result in functional improvement sometime in the future,[14] but the future is now. Palisano said, "in the present climate of health care reform, the extent that consumers identify our services as being responsive to their needs will impact greatly on how well we will be positioned to face the challenges of the 21st century."[38(p140)] This is true regardless of the service setting and who pays for the services.

CONCLUSION

For a long time, special education has fostered measurable functional goals, teaching approaches that promote learning and generalization, and parental involvement. The current direction of pediatric therapy clearly supports these special education tenets. Systems-based theories of motor behavior, motor learning principles, disablement models, and family-centered practices have not only strengthened the links between special education and pediatric therapy, but they have blurred distinctions between "educational therapy" and "medical therapy."

Whether the team is comprised of a parent, child, and therapist, or consists of a roomful of family and school professionals, the team's job is to identify functional goals that are meaningful to the family and child, determine sound means to accomplish them, decide upon environments for teaching and learning, and identify as many opportunities for practice as possible. The effectiveness of the intervention must then be measured by the child's accomplishment of the functional goals. These functional goals are the child's goals, not medical therapy goals or educational therapy goals. Depending on what the parents and the rest of the educational team determine the child's educational priorities to be, goals requiring therapy as a related service in an educational environment and goals of intervention in a medical setting could be identical.

REFERENCES

1. Education for All Handicapped Children Act of 1975. (Public Law 94-142), 20 U.S.C. S1401.

2. Heriza CB: Pediatric physical therapy: reflections of the past and visions for the future. *Pediatr Phys Ther.* 1994; 6: 105-106.

3. Heriza CB, Sweeney JK: Pediatric physical therapy: part I. Practice scope, scientific basis, and theoretical foundation. *Inf Young Children.* 1994; 7(2): 20-32.

4. Horak FB: Assumptions underlying motor control for neurologic rehabilitation. In: Lister MJ, ed. *Contemporary Management of Motor Control Problems: Proceedings of the II Step Conference.* Alexandria, VA: Foundation for Physical Therapy; 1991: 11-27.

5. Stuberg W, Harbourne R: Theoretical practice in pediatric physical therapy: past, present, and future considerations. *Pediatr Phys Ther.* 1994; 6: 119-125.

6. Case-Smith J, Fisher AG, Bauer D: An analysis of the relationship between proximal and distal motor control. *Am J Occup Ther.* 1989; 43: 657-662.

7. Horowitz L, Sharby N: Development of prone extension postures in healthy infants. *Phys Ther.* 1988; 68: 32-39.

8. Thelen E: Rhythmical stereotypies in normal human infants. *Animal Behavior.* 1979; 27: 699-715.

9. Kamm J, Thelen E, Jensen J: A dynamical systems approach to motor development. *Phys Ther.* 1990; 70: 763-775.

10. Bradley NS: Motor control: developmental aspects of motor control in skill acquisition. In: Campbell SK, ed. *Physical Therapy for Children.* Philadelphia, PA: WB Saunders; 1994: 39-77.

11. Haley SM, Baryza MJ, Blanchard Y: Functional and naturalistic frameworks in assessing physical and motor disablement. In: Wilhelm IJ, ed. *Physical Therapy Assessment in Early Infancy.* New York, NY: Churchill Livingstone; 1993: 225-256.

12. Heriza C: Motor development: traditional and contemporary theories. In: Lister MJ, ed. *Contemporary Management of Motor Control Problems: Proceedings of the II STEP Conference.* Alexandria, VA: Foundation for Physical Therapy; 1991: 99-126.

13. Shumway-Cook A, Woollacott M: *Motor Control: Theory and Practical Applications.* Baltimore, MD: Williams & Wilkins; 1995.

14. Gordon J: Assumptions underlying physical therapy intervention: theoretical and historical perspectives. In: Carr JH, Shepherd RB, eds. *Movement Science: Foundations for Physical Therapy in Rehabilitation.* Rockville, MD: Aspen Publishers; 1987: 1-30.

15. Harris SR, McEwen IR: Assessing motor skills. In: McLean ML, Bailey D, Wolery M, eds. *Assessing Infants and Toddlers with Special Needs.* Columbus, OH: Merrill; in press.

16. Schmidt RA: Motor learning principles for physical therapy. In: *Lister MJ, ed. Contemporary Management of Motor Control Problems: Proceedings of the II STEP Conference.* Alexandria, VA: Foundation for Physical Therapy; 1991: 49-62.

17. Mulligan M, Lacy L, Guess D: Effects of massed, distributed or spaced trial sequencing on severely handicapped students' performance. *J Assoc Sev Handicap.* 1982; 7(2): 48-61.

18. Snell ME, Zirpoli TJ: Intervention strategies. In: Snell ME, ed. *Systematic Instruction of Persons with Severe Handicaps.* 3rd ed. Columbus, OH: Charles E Merrill; 1987: 110-149.

19. Haring NG: *Generalization for Students with Severe Handicaps.* University of Washington, Seattle, WA: Washington Research Organization; 1988.

20. Stokes TF, Baer DL: An implicit technology of generalization. *J of Appl Behav Analysis.* 1977; 10; 349-367.

21. Shea JB, Morgan RL: Contextual interference effects on the acquisition, retention, and transfer of a motor skill. *J Exp Psychol [Hum Learn Mem].* 1979; 5: 179-187.

22. Man AM, Adams JA, Donchin E: Adaptive and part-whole training in the acquisition of a complex perceptual-motor skill. *Acta Psychol (Amst).* 1989; 71: 179-196.

23. Winstein CJ: Designing practice for motor learning: clinical implications. In: *Lister MJ, ed. Contemporary Management of Motor Control Problems: Proceedings of the II STEP Conference.* Alexandria, VA: Foundation for Physical Therapy; 1991: 65-76.

24. Kaplan M: Motor learning: implications for occupational therapy and neurodevelopmental treatment. *Developmental Disabilities Special Interest Section Newsletter.* 1994; 17(3): 1-4.

25. Jette AM: Physical disablement concepts for physical therapy research and practice. *Phys Ther.* 1994; 74: 380-386.

26. Nagi S: Some conceptual issues in disability and rehabilitation. In: Sussman M, ed. *Sociology and Rehabilitation.* Washington, DC: American Sociological Association: 1965; 100-113.

27. *International Classification of Impairments, Disabilities, and Handicaps.* Geneva, Switzerland: World Health Organization; 1980.

28. Haley SM, Coster WJ, Ludlow LH, Haltiwanger JT, Andrellos PJ: *Pediatric Evaluation of Disability Inventory (PEDI): Development, Standardization and Administration Manual.* Boston, MA: New England Medical Center Hospitals; 1992.

29. Campbell SK, Vander Linden DW, Palisano RJ, eds. *Physical Therapy for Children.* Philadelphia, PA: WB Saunders; 1994.

30. *Research Plan for the National Center for Medical Rehabilitation Research.* U.S. Department of Health and Human Services; 1993.

31. Harris SR: Early intervention: does developmental therapy make a difference? *Topics in Early Childhood Special Education.* 1988; 7(4): 20-32.

32. Russell D, Rosenbaum P, Gowland C et al: *Gross Motor Function Measure.* Hamilton, Ontario, Canada: Gross Motor Measures Group; 1990.

33. Campbell PH: Evaluation and assessment in early intervention for infants and toddlers. *Journal of Early Intervention.* 1991; 15: 36-45.

34. Dunn W: Measurement of function: actions for the future. *Am J Occup Ther.* 1992; 47: 357-359.

35. Folio MR, Fewell RR: *Peabody Developmental Motor Scales and Activity Cards.* Chicago, IL: Riverside Publishing; 1983.

36. Payton OD, Nelson CE, Ozer MN: *Patient Participation in Program Planning: A Manual for Therapists.* Philadelphia, PA: FA Davis Company; 1990.

37. Education of the Handicapped Act Amendments of 1986. (Public Law 99-457), 20 U.S.C. S1400.

38. Palisano RJ: Pediatric physical therapy: an individual perspective. *Pediatr Phys Ther.* 1994; 6: 140-141.

Related Services Decision-Making:
A Foundational Component
of Effective Education
for Students with Disabilities

Michael F. Giangreco

SUMMARY. This article presents a variety of issues pertaining to how decisions are made about educationally related services for students with disabilities. The first section discusses areas of general agreement in the field, as well as challenges, associated with the current state-of-the-art in related service decision-making. The second major section of the article highlights a series of guidelines that offer alternatives believed to address some of the limitations associated with current practices. Topics include: (a) teamwork; (b) defining

Michael F. Giangreco, PhD, is Research Assistant Professor, College of Education and Social Services, The University Affiliated Program of Vermont, 499C Waterman Building, University of Vermont, Burlington, VT 05405.

Partial support for the preparation of this manuscript was provided by the United States Department of Education, Office of Special Education and Rehabilitative Services under the category, Research Validation and Implementation Projects for Children Who Are Deaf-Blind, CFDA 84.0258 (HO25S40003), awarded to the University Affiliated Program of Vermont at the University of Vermont. The contents of this paper reflect the ideas and positions of the author and do not necessarily reflect the ideas or positions of the U.S. Department of Education, therefore no official endorsement should be inferred.

This article is based on portions of the *Vermont Independent Service Team Approach: A Guide to Coordinating Educational Support Services*, written by the author, Burlington, VT, University of Vermont, College of Education.

[Haworth co-indexing entry note]: "Related Services Decision-Making: A Foundational Component of Effective Education for Students with Disabilities." Giangreco, Michael F. Co-published simultaneously in *Physical & Occupational Therapy in Pediatrics* (The Haworth Press, Inc.) Vol. 15, No. 2, 1995, pp. 47-67; and: *Occupational and Physical Therapy in Educational Environments* (ed: Irene R. McEwen) The Haworth Press, Inc., 1995, pp. 47-67. Single or multiple copies of this article are available from The Haworth Document Delivery Service [1-800-342-9678, 9:00 a.m - 5:00 p.m. (EST)].

educational program components; (c) the relationship between program, placement, and services; (d) values that underlie decision-making; (e) functions of related services; (f) criteria for related service decision-making; (g) decision-making authority practices; (h) modes of service provision; (i) location and strategies for service provision; and (j) implementation and evaluation of related services. *[Article copies available from The Haworth Document Delivery Service: 1-800-342-9678.]*

It is generally acknowledged that the provision of educationally related services, such as occupational therapy and physical therapy, are important for many students with disabilities to have access to education and adequately participate in their educational program, including pursuit of identified learning outcomes. How is the need for related services determined? How are decisions made about the frequency of service provision? How is it determined whether services will be provided directly by the therapist or indirectly, on a consultative basis, through another team member? These and other critical service provision and coordination questions typically have been left to professionals to answer, based on their own personal and clinical judgment. The purpose of this article is two-fold. First, issues pertaining to the current status of related services are presented. This introductory section discusses areas of general agreement in the field as well as challenges associated with the current state-of-the-art in related service decision-making. The second major section of the article highlights a series of guidelines that offer alternatives believed to address some of the limitations associated with current practices.

SOME CURRENT ISSUES IN RELATED SERVICES

Almost without exception, the literature and litigation pertaining to the provision of related services for students with disabilities in schools (e.g., physical therapy, occupational therapy, speech/language pathology, orientation/mobility) mention that related services must, ". . . be required to assist a child with disability to benefit from special education . . ." as originally stipulated by P.L. 94-142 *(Education for All Handicapped Children Act of 1975)* and subsequently by P.L. 101-476 *(Individuals with Disabilities Education Act of 1990).*[1-16] For students whose unique characteristics require knowledge and skills beyond those typically possessed by teachers, related services can be crucial in developing and implementing an appropriately individualized educational program. Yet the literature also presents a long-standing concern that groups formed by educational and related service professionals often function in disjointed and fragmented ways, thus highlighting the need for more collaborative relationships.[5,17-21] The mere presence of many professionals from a variety of disciplines, regardless of each person's individual competencies, does not ensure that students will receive educationally relevant and necessary related services. Ultimately, the education of students with disabilities is compromised when input from a related service professional is not adequately synthesized with the input of the family, educational staff, and other related service providers.

Services are more likely to be *disjointed and fragmented when professionals do not share the common conceptual tenet that related services are required to be educationally relevant and necessary.* Many skillful and well-intentioned related service providers are still trained and professionally socialized to function independently within their discipline rather than interdependently as a member of a collaborative educational team. Despite all the rhetoric about teamwork, too many professionals still assess, plan, make service provision decisions, implement, and evaluate in relative isolation. Evidence collected from 585 professionals and parents across the country highlighted a series of common professional practices that respondents reported they engaged in frequently; these practices are likely to interfere with the integrated provision of related services.[22] For example, respondents indicated that it was a common practice for related service professionals to make decisions about issues such as the need for related services, frequency of service, and mode of provision (e.g., direct, indirect) prior to knowing the student's IEP (individualized education plan) goals. Educationally relevant and necessary related service recommendations cannot be made purposefully if one does not first know the contents of the educational program as reflected, in part, by the IEP. In many schools it is not uncommon for a person from each related service discipline to generate a separate set of goals which reflect outcomes valued by the respective discipline. Not only can this be confusing for families, it creates a problem whereby group members agree to each pursue discipline-specific goals rather than sharing a set of educational goals that are discipline-free; in essence group members may reach consensus to head in different directions. Examples from a recent study of 47 IEPs of students with multiple disabilities documented numerous examples where separate goals were listed by professional disciplines.[23] This raises serious questions about whether team members shared a common framework to pursue the educational relevance and necessity of service provision.

A second major problem resulting in disjointed and fragmented services is *ambiguous roles and expectations among service providers* working with the same child.[24] In a workshop activity I have conducted with thousands of educators, related service providers, and parents across the country, ambiguous roles and disorganization consistently have been selected as the two most prominent forms of group dysfunction. Additionally, a recent study[25] demonstrated that educators, parents, and related service providers differ regarding who should have authority for making related service decisions. The study showed that related service providers strongly favored retaining decision authority regarding their own discipline; both special educators and parents whose children have disabilities favored consensus decision-making instead. Such potential ambiguity and differing expectations present fertile ground for conflicts among team members and for due process hearings.

Existing models for making related service decisions, most of which lack research support, are designed to assist in sorting out issues such as the type, frequency, and mode of service provision (e.g., direct, consult), yet these models may actually contribute to the fragmentation of services. Many professionals anxious for seemingly logical and expedient ways to make complicated decisions, are drawn to existing decision-models which may have some positive features, but tend to share a common conceptual orientation that often is not recognized as problematic.[1,26-29] These models examine decision-making exclusively from the perspective of a single discipline such as occupational therapy or physical therapy.[30] Such unidisciplinary decision-making models do not account for the fact that many of the functions served by educational team members from various disciplines can, and do, overlap with those of other disciplines. A unidisciplinary orientation limits an individual team member's ability to make educationally relevant related service decisions as required by the *Individuals with Disabilities Education Act of 1990* because it fails to address the interrelationships among the disciplines involved in a student's education. When professionals make related service decisions in a unidisciplinary fashion, based on what they individually value from the perspective of their own disciplines, there is an increased probability of undesirable and unnecessary overlaps and gaps in services, contradictory recommendations from service providers, and conflicts among team members; unidisciplinary decision-making likely perpetuates role ambiguity and programmatic fragmentation.

Although these issues are sufficiently important to warrant action to improve the provision of educationally related services, another major factor compounds the challenge. Traditionally, students with multiple and/ or severe disabilities, presumably those receiving the most extensive related services, have been educated in special education classes and schools. Related service providers working in these settings often were encouraged, or asked directly by educational administrators or teachers, to generate separate goals, independently make service provision decisions, and provide direct services in isolated settings despite the fact that these practices violate the tenets of collaborative teamwork. Over the past few years new opportunities have become available for increasing numbers of students with disabilities, including those with multiple and/or severe disabilities, to be educated in general education classes while pursuing either the general education program with suitable access accommodations or a modified/individualized program with supports.[31]

Although the literature highlights many problems regarding related service provision, clearly there have been, and are, many examples where related service providers, educators, and families have worked together effectively to support students with disabilities. On the other hand, some well-intentioned professionals have attempted to transfer positive features of support from traditional, disability-only, settings to general education schools and classes. This generally does not work well because the contextual differences among classes and schools serving only students with disabilities and those serving a heterogeneous population consisting primarily of children without disabilities are so vast.[32] Just because something was valued, made sense, and seemed to work in one context does not mean it will be valued, make sense, and work in another context.

As we move further into this new era of opportunities for students with and without disabilities to be educated together, the time is right to establish the importance of effective coordination and provision of educationally relevant and necessary related services. Programmatic advances and research pertaining to related service decision-making, provision, and effectiveness will continue to be a critical need because:

a. such services affect a high proportion of students with disabilities in public schools across every age group and racial/cultural heritage;
b. the involvement of professionals from various disciplines is considered both necessary and desirable in supporting the education of many students with disabilities,[4,33] yet existing, invalidated approaches suffer from a unidisciplinary orientation resulting in gaps, overlaps, contradictions, and role ambiguity among service providers;
c. the literature indicates that cross-disciplinary service relationships pose currently unresolved problems related to coordination and decision-making among professionals and between professionals and families whose children have disabilities, resulting in disjointed and fragmented educational programs;[5,18-20,34]

    d. insufficient research data exist regarding related services to draw empirically sound conclusions regarding their effectiveness in supporting the education of students with disabilities;[35]

    e. the national movement to include more students in general education schools and classrooms is raising new issues regarding appropriate service provision as the context for service provision shifts to educational settings frequented predominantly by students without disabilities;[32,36]

    f. the shift toward general education placements has resulted in a shift in staffing patterns from related service providers as employees of special schools or health agencies, to related service providers as private contractors and/or school district employees; this has altered the role of related service providers and their relationship to local education agencies and school personnel in ways that have yet to be studied or fully understood;

    g. with the passage of P.L. 99-457 and its emphasis on service provision in the least restrictive environments, increasing numbers of young children with disabilities are making the transition from early intervention programs into integrated daycare settings, preschools, and kindergartens, thus adding to our need to understand related service issues more thoroughly and develop approaches to serve students and families more effectively; and

    h. families and people with disabilities are increasingly expressing concern about the transition from school to community living and the critical need for related service type supports after graduation in terms of living arrangements, work, transportation, recreation, and communication access.[37-40]

ALTERNATIVE PRINCIPLES TO GUIDE
RELATED SERVICE DECISION-MAKING

The following subsections describe ten interrelated guidelines that provide alternative ways to think about related service provision in educational settings (see Table 1). These interrelated guidelines have been applied to the practice of related service decision-making through a process known as VISTA (Vermont Interdependent Services Team Approach).[18,41] Specific instructions for the use of VISTA are beyond the scope of this article. Although VISTA represents one way of organizing these guidelines, their applicability is not limited to use within the VISTA framework–they can be valuable guidelines and principles when used less systematically and can likely be organized in a variety of ways to support reasoned, collaborative decision-making.

TABLE 1. Interrelated Guidelines to Facilitate Related Service Decision-Making

1. Establish and Maintain a Collaborative Team

2. Define Components of the Educational Program

3. Understand the Interaction Among Program, Placement and Services

4. Use a Value System to Guide Decision-Making: "Only-As-Special-As-Necessary"

5. Determine Functions of Service Providers and Their Interrelatedness

6. Apply Essential Criteria When Making Service Recommendations: Educational Relevance and Necessity

7. Determine Who Has Authority for Decision-Making: Consensus

8. Match the Mode and Frequency of Service Provision to the Function Served

9. Determine the Least Restrictive Location and Strategies for Service Provision

10. Implement and Evaluate Related Services

When used in combination, these guidelines are designed to: (a) increase team members' confidence that their related service provision decisions are educationally relevant and necessary; (b) increase reliability among a team regarding which aspects of a student's program require support from various members and what functions those members need to serve (who is doing what to whom and why); (c) reduce unnecessary and undesirable overlaps, gaps, and contradictions in related service provision recommendations; (d) reduce conflicts among team members by focusing intra-team communication on student- and context-specific information; (e) assist in matching the mode and frequency of service provision to the functions of related service involvement required to support an individual student's educational program; (f) guide implementation of related services in supportive but minimally intrusive ways; (g) evaluate services based on learning outcomes and valued life outcomes; and (h) increase team members' satisfaction with their related service decision-making practices. Initial research on VISTA with six student planning teams serving students with multiple disabilities has yielded promising results;[18] a series of additional studies are underway. The following sections summarize some of the main points pertaining to the ten interrelated guidelines we find to be useful when making educationally relevant and necessary related service decisions.

Establish and Maintain a Collaborative Team

Although having two or more members is essential to establishing and maintaining a collaborative team, it is not sufficient, even if the members possess various skills and knowledge, share information, and regularly meet together. First, we must ensure that the members of the team include those people who will be affected by decisions made by the team.[42] In addition to special educators and related service providers who are typically part of the team, it is critical to include the student when appropriate, the parents, general education teachers, paraprofessionals, and potentially others (e.g., peers, bus drivers, administrators). In some cases, on the other hand, the number of team members can become overwhelming and make decision-making unnecessarily complicated. A recent study of students with multiple disabilities indicated team sizes ranging from 5 to 21 with the average team including 11 members.[23] Teams can reduce the number of people involved in regular meetings by designating a *core* team comprised of those people who have the most ongoing involvement with the student and an *extended* team that includes the core team plus those members who have less frequent involvement with the student, and by establishing *situational* teams comprised of individually determined combinations of team members to address specific issues or concerns. In this way, team members' time can be used efficiently.

Once team membership has been established, the most foundational and defining characteristic that distinguishes a *collection of people* from a *team* is the development of a shared framework and the purposeful pursuit of a shared or common set of goals. Important supportive characteristics of teamwork, such as sharing resources, effective communication, and consensus decision-making, ultimately will only have the desired impact when applied within a shared framework and to meet common goals.

Define Components of the Educational Program

One of the most explicit ways to operationalize a shared framework and common goals is for the team to reach agreement and document the components of a student's educational program. The framework discussed here for determining the components of the educational program is based on COACH (Choosing Options and Accommodations for CHildren).[43] The components of the educational program can be broadly categorized as a student's: (a) priority learning outcomes, (b) additional learning outcomes, and (c) general supports; these components describe only *what* the educational program will consist of and do not address issues of where or how education will be provided.

A student's *priority learning outcomes* refer to a small set of the most important learning outcomes. These priority learning outcomes are family selected, individualized, and discipline-free. They are not based on what is valued from the perspective of various disciplines, but rather are referenced to individually determined valued life outcomes, such as personal health, having personally meaningful social relationships, having age-appropriate choice and control, having access to personally and societally valued places and activities, developing skills for life-long learning, and contributing to one's community. Priority learning outcomes typically are documented as annual goals and short-term objectives on the IEP.

Additional learning outcomes refer to individually determined student program content that extends beyond the small set and potentially narrow boundaries of the top priorities. These additional learning outcomes, determined jointly by team members, are designed to ensure that the student has access to a broad range of learning outcomes from curriculum areas included in the general education program as well as other sources that extend beyond it in any direction. For example, if a particular student's priority learning outcomes focus primarily on communication, social, and self-care areas, additional learning outcomes may include other items from those same areas as well as learning outcomes from different curriculum areas, such as language arts, math, science, physical education, arts, or computer literacy. The configuration and number of additional learning outcomes will vary for each student based on his or her individual needs and characteristics.

The third category, which completes the components of the educational program, are *general supports* that *need to be provided to or for the student* to allow access to education or to facilitate participation in the educational program. Unlike the learning outcomes discussed in the previous paragraphs which seek observable changes in student behavior, general supports seek changes in the behavior of team members other than the student. General supports generally are broad and cross-situational as opposed to highly specific to a particular lesson. Five categories of general supports have been listed in COACH; they include: (a) *personal needs* (e.g., feeding, dressing, giving medication); (b) *physical needs* (e.g., therapeutic positioning, managing specialized equipment, environmental modifications); (c) *sensory needs* (e.g., Braille translation, access to large print materials, sign language interpretation); (d) *teaching others about the student* (e.g., teaching classmates the student's augmentative communication system; teaching staff crisis intervention or health emergency protocols); and (e) *providing access and opportunities* (e.g., arranging community-based vocational experiences, providing literacy materials in the student's native language, providing access to regular class activities).

Explicitly documenting the components of a student's educational program in this way has at least three primary benefits. First, the agreed upon set of learning outcomes and general supports become the basis for determining the educational relevance of related services; decision-making would be compromised if team members agree to this shared list yet retain a separate agenda of learning outcomes and general supports. Second, clearly differentiating between learning outcomes and general supports provides clear expectations regarding what we expect the student to learn and do versus what we expect other team members to learn and do. Unnecessary conflicts arise when team members have different expectations about educational program components. For example, one member may be under the impression that the student is learning dressing skills and wheelchair transfers, while another thought these were supports for the student. Third, research has indicated that professionals sometimes confuse learning outcomes and general supports so that IEP annual goals are actually general supports rather than learning outcomes–this can result in IEPs that are unnecessarily passive and therefore do not tap the learning potential of students.[23,44] "Rosa will be repositioned every half hour" is an example of a general support that may need to be provided for Rosa but positioning is not an annual goal that requires Rosa to learn.

Understand the Interaction Among Program, Placement, and Services

Existing data[22] suggest that the sequence with which professionals consider a student's program, placement, and services may interfere with developing an appropriately individualized program in the least restrictive environment. For example, evidence suggests that related services providers frequently make service decisions in isolation prior to knowing the educational program components, thus making the educational relevance and necessity of such services unknown. In some cases, professionals reported recommending placement of a student in special education school so he or she could get access to related services, also prior to knowing the educational program components. Although both of these scenarios are common practice, they reflect questionable logic because such service recommendations are likely based on presumed disability characteristics rather than individually identified needs.

The sequence of program, then placement, then services is offered here as an approach that is conceptually, philosophically, and pragmatically congruent with the intent to have related services be educationally relevant and necessary. By determining the educational program components first, we know what we want the student to learn and experience in school. Once we know what we want for the student, based on his or her individual needs, we can then consider the least restrictive placement option where the student can pursue the identified educational program components. The *Individuals with Disabilities Education Act of 1990* along with the 1994 decision in the California case of Sacramento City Unified School District v. Rachel H.[45] have reaffirmed that the general education classroom is the primary placement option for students with disabilities, including those with the most severe disabilities. It is crucial to remember that the law states that a student should only be removed from regular class if his or her individual needs cannot be met when given supplemental supports and aids; it does not say that students should be denied access to the regular class based on categorical disability labels, their need for individualized curriculum and/ or instruction within the general class setting, or their need for specialized supports. Determination of related service needs logically comes after determining educational program components and placement because the latter factors will influence the need for related services.

Use a Value System to Guide Decision-Making: "Only-As-Special-As-Necessary"

Decision-making models are all based on underlying assumptions and values which are sometimes clearly articulated for the consumer and other times require a bit of detective work to figure out. Exemplary practices in education and related services are rooted in a broad set of values, such as access, equity, individualization, interdependence, diversity, collaboration, and community.[46] Given the enormous variation that exists among students, families, schools, and communities, having an underlying value system can assist team members when faced with unique challenges by facilitating consideration of whether the decisions and actions being proposed are congruent or incongruent with the team's underlying values.

When specifically considering related service decision-making, some team members practice a "more-is-better" approach. Like the young child who would rather have ten pennies than one quarter, this approach is misguided because it confuses quantity with value. Another, hopefully less prevalent, approach is "return-on-investment" which places a high value on serving students who have a favorable history and prognosis for being remediated and those likely to contribute the most, economically, to society. Return-on-investment approaches fail to recognize the important contributions made by people with the most severe disabilities that may be difficult to measure in dollars and cents. Parents have concerns that professionals may use the "return-on-investment" approach as a rationale for reducing or discontinuing services to a student rather than risk exposing that they are challenged by a situation and may not know exactly what to do.[34] This parental observation raises important and difficult questions that we must ask ourselves as professionals. It is heartening to note that the same set of parents preferred that professionals honestly acknowledge when they do not know something and be willing to support needs identified by families. Theoretically, the pressures to guard one's professionalism by avoiding challenging situations can be reduced when we support each other within a collaborative team.

An alternative value system that allows for various combinations of direct and indirect services is to provide supports that are "only-as-special-as-necessary."[47,48] This approach allows for the provision of needed services and acknowledges the contributions made by various disciplines, but takes precautions to avoid the inherent drawbacks of well-intentioned over service. Providing more services than are necessary may: (a) decrease time for participation in activities with non-disabled peers; (b) cause disruption in acquiring, practicing, or generalizing other important educational skills; (c) cause inequities in the distribution of scarce resources when some students in need remain unserved or underserved; (d) overwhelm families with the involvement of an unnecessarily high number of professionals; (e) create unnecessary or unhealthy dependencies; or (f) unnecessarily complicate communication and coordination among team members. The "only-as-special-as-necessary" approach is based on the notion that rather than trying to obtain the *most* services possible, we should seek to determine the appropriate amount and type of services for each individual student, not too little, not too much; this will necessarily be a collective "best guess."

Determine Functions of Service Providers and Their Interrelatedness

It is critical for team members to have a shared understanding of what functions each person is serving and how they interrelate to support the student's educational program. In a recent study, 318 special educators, related service providers, and parents of students with severe disabilities rated a set of related service functions commonly cited in the professional literature.[25] These people indicated that the four most important functions for serving students with severe disabilities were: (a) developing adaptations and/or equipment to allow for active participation and/or prevent negative outcomes (e.g., regression, deformity, discomfort, pain); (b) transferring information and skills to others (e.g., related service providers, educators, parents); (c) serving as a resource and/or support to the family; and (d) applying discipline-specific methods or techniques to promote active participation and/or prevent negative outcomes. These essential functions may be augmented by discretionary functions that are individually and situationally appropriate.[25] Clarifying the functions served by each team member and the interrelatedness of these functions helps to further develop the team's shared framework and allows members to purposely explore service functions for potential gaps, overlaps, and contradictions.

Apply Essential Criteria When Making Service Recommendations: Educational Relevance and Necessity

The professional literature is replete with suggested criteria for making related service decisions for students with disabilities.[1,26-29] Some of the criteria are situationally useful and others highly suspect; only two appear to be essential across all situations. First, we must always consider whether a proposed related service is *educationally relevant*. We can do this by referencing it to identified components of the student's individual educational program as previously identified by the team. If the proposed related service is relevant to the educational program, then we must employ the second essential criterion to determine whether the related service is *necessary*.

There are at least four basic ways to test for educational necessity. First, we can ask ourselves if there are any existing data or logic to suggest that the absence of the proposed service will interfere with the student's access to or participation in his or her educational program, including pursuit of identified learning outcomes. If the absence of the service poses a threat to access or meaningful participation, then the service is necessary; if it does not pose such a threat, it is not necessary. Making such decisions requires team members to rely on the "only-as-special-as-necessary" value system. If the service passes this test for necessity, we can then consider potential gaps, overlaps, and contradictions among team members. For example, a necessary service to provide appropriate therapeutic positioning could be suggested by both the occupational therapist and the physical therapist. Team members need to clarify what they are referring to regarding therapeutic positioning; if members' skills are overlapping, the team needs to decide whether the overlap is necessary and desirable or not. A third way to explore the potential necessity of related services is to check with both the sender and receiver of the service. For example, an occupational therapist may say that she needs to serve the function of transferring specialized information and skills regarding eating and drinking to the paraprofessional who works with the student at lunch time. In this example, although serving this function may meet the previously suggested tests for necessity, the team members may agree that the paraprofessional is sufficiently experienced and skilled with this particular student that such support is not necessary. In an opposite scenario, the potential receiver of a service can make it known that he or she needs a certain type of support. For example, if the general supports for a student indicate that one of the student's personal needs is assistance with eating, the teacher may raise the fact that the newly hired paraprofessional has no experience assisting a child with oral-motor difficulties with eating and therefore may require transfer of information and skills from the occupational therapist. When possible, it is always desirable to check directly with the student; this can provide essential information and promote self-advocacy. A fourth test for necessity is to consider whether a service provided in one context can be adequately generalized to other settings without the direct involvement of the specialist. For example, if the physical therapist has assisted core team members by sharing specialized information and skills pertaining to transfers in and out of a student's wheelchair in the general education classroom, the team needs to determine whether it is necessary for the therapist to be directly involved in the same transfer of information and skills across all environments where wheelchair transfers will occur (e.g., gymnasium, cafeteria, playground, library) or whether such information and skills can be adequately transferred to other places and people, possibly with the specialist monitoring periodically to ensure quality and accountability. Use of these simple tests of necessity can assist in avoiding the inherent problems of over service discussed earlier.

Determine Who Has Authority for Decision-Making: Consensus

Three basic options exist for making decisions; autocratic, democratic, and consensus.[25] Each possesses positive and negative features. In autocratic decision-making, the specialist retains individual authority. Democratic decision-making provides one vote for each team member, and like an election, majority rules. Both autocratic and democratic decision-making are quick, easy, and familiar, but they have drawbacks. Autocratic decision-making increases the probability of individual errors in judgment and is likely to perpetuate disjointed and fragmented services by failing to account for interrelationships with other team members. This issue can become especially problematic for school-based staff when well-intentioned physicians write prescriptions for services like occupational therapy and physical therapy without the benefit of being part of the team or having any notion of the educational relevance and/or necessity of the services they are prescribing. Democratic decision-making tends to polarize factions within teams, fails to recognize the potential value of dissenting opinions, and invariably leaves parents outnumbered.

Although consensus decision-making is likely to require more time and effort than autocratic or democratic approaches, the benefits of this option outweigh the drawbacks. By reaching mutually valued agreements, team members strengthen and extend the development of their shared framework, have opportunities to learn from and support each other, and establish clearly communicated expectations designed to facilitate effective service provision and quality education.

Match the Mode of Service Provision to the Functions Served

For years the professional literature has included debates about the virtues and pitfalls of direct versus indirect/consultative service provision. The issue is not which mode of service provision is better, but rather which mode or combination of modes matches the function being served. Once a function (e.g., making an adapted switch for use of a communication device) has been determined to be educationally relevant (by being referenced to an identified component of a student's educational program) and educationally necessary, the appropriate mode(s) of service provision can be selected by considering whether the function lends itself to direct or indirect service. For example, let's assume that an occupational therapist builds or modifies the adapted switch so that it is individually appropriate for the student and then trains other team members on its use. Both of these functions (making the adaptation and transferring information/skills) are indirect services. These indirect functions require the specialist to have knowledge of the student and interact with him, but the purpose of that interaction is to gather information and/or work through others rather than to provide direct therapeutic intervention. It is conceivable that a student could receive educationally relevant and necessary related services indirectly or through a direct/indirect combination. Because the skills and knowledge of related service providers need to be extended to other team members, it is almost inconceivable that a student could receive appropriate related services in a direct service mode exclusively, yet this remains a common practice. Team members can determine which mode(s) of service provision match the functions determined to be educationally relevant and necessary and then can make an initial "best guess" at how much time will be required to fulfill the identified functions. Be wary of formulas that offer prescribed modes of service provision and/or suggested frequencies and duration of service; there are simply too many unique variables about students, families, team members, schools, and communities for such formulas to offer appropriate individualization. Reasoned decision-making will be aided by a group of competent and caring team members working together to understand each others' perspectives and building a shared framework.

Determine the Least Restrictive Location
and Strategies for Service Provision

Traditionally, many related services have been provided in isolated settings such as therapy rooms using specialized strategies that may be considered unusual or intrusive if used in general classroom settings. As integrated provision of related services became increasingly recognized as more effective than isolated service provision, confusion surfaced regarding where and how these new integrated services were to occur.[49,50] Some well-intentioned team members arranged for traditional, isolated therapy to take place within the classroom; this does *not* necessarily constitute integrated provision of related services. In fact, provision of certain types of service in the classroom or other school locations could potentially be quite inappropriate. For example, one day in a school cafeteria, a concerned second-grader asked me, "Why does that lady have Lauren in a headlock and why is she making her gag–I don't think Lauren is having a very good time." An itinerant occupational therapist was attempting to elicit a gag reflex and subsequently was using full jaw control with Lauren. Although the techniques used by the therapist are rather standard and would not stand out negatively in a special school or special class, in the general education cafeteria they appeared more like a combination of Championship Wrestling and some sort of punishment than techniques designed to be helpful.

Team members should strive to provide services in the most natural environments and use approaches that are socially acceptable within those integrated settings. As mentioned earlier, when contexts change, we must realize that other people's reality may be different from our own. What we do for, or with, students with disabilities must enhance their status. In other words we need to make sure that we do not make students with disabilities look bad in front of their peers in the name of "service." It is important to consider the student's privacy, dignity, and the perceptions of peers when selecting both where services will be provided and what strategies will be used. If the team agrees for some individualized reason that a student temporarily needs to receive services in a private setting (as might be true for a student without disabilities), plans should be put in place to monitor the situation and create mechanisms to re-integrate the student into the typical school and classroom settings as soon as possible. When considering location and strategies, always start with and strive for those that are the least restrictive and least intrusive while attending to identified student needs.

Implement and Evaluate Related Services

Once the team has thought through a reasoned plan, related services can be implemented either through a combination of direct and indirect services or through primarily indirect services. One question often left unanswered is whether the provision of the related service has been effective. The first step in being able to evaluate the impact of a related service is to know what components of the educational program the service was intended to support. As discussed earlier in this article, the related service could be designed to address the student's learning outcomes or general supports. By knowing which educational program components are being supported and which functions are being served, the team can ask individually appropriate questions such as: (a) Has the service provided access to, or allowed for participation in, the educational program? or (b) Has the service facilitated improvement in identified learning that would probably not occur in the absence of the service? Although educational access, participation, and improvement in learning outcomes are meaningful indicators of related service effectiveness, ultimately the team must consider if, and how, the student has experienced positive changes in his or her valued life outcomes as a result of the service. In other words, is the student's life better and, if so, how, as a result of receiving this service? Thinking about these kinds of quality of life issues is complex and highly individualized.[51] Parents of children with disabilities have identified some valued life outcomes as: (a) being safe and healthy; (b) having networks of personally meaningful relationships; (c) having choice and control that matches one's age; (d) having a variety of interesting places to go and meaningful activities to do; (e) having a home to live in, now and in the future; (f) engaging in personal growth and lifelong learning; and (g) contributing to one's community.[34,52] Are not these the same outcomes that many families value for their children who do not have disability labels? As we gather both quantitative and qualitative data to evaluate the impact of related services, we are challenged to continually cycle through the process of considering the educational relevance and necessity of services and the emergent interrelationships among team members as changes occur in team membership, the context for learning, the family, and the student.

CONCLUSION

This article has presented a series of ideas designed to assist you in considering the related service needs of students with disabilities as they increasingly access typical school and other community environments along with people who do not have disabilities. Given the history of related services decision-making and provision in public schools, the need for further research and programmatic advances is evident. Therefore, the ideas presented here are meant as a springboard to continue cross-disciplinary discussions designed to serve students with disabilities and their families more effectively.

AUTHOR NOTE

The author wishes to acknowledge and thank Irene McEwen and Beverly Rainforth for their helpful editing suggestions during the preparation of this manuscript.

REFERENCES

1. American Occupational Therapy Association: *Guidelines for Occupational Therapy Services in School Systems* (second edition). Rockville, MD: American Occupational Therapy Association; 1989.

2. American Physical Therapy Association: *APTA Guidelines for Physical Therapy Practice in Education Environments*. Alexandria, VA: American Physical Therapy Association; 1989.

3. *Board of Education of the Hendrick Hudson Central School v. Rowley*, 102 S. Ct 3034, 1982.

4. Campbell PH: The integrated programming team: An approach for coordinating professionals of various disciplines in programs for students with severe and multiple handicaps. *Journal of the Association for Persons with Severe Handicaps.* 1987; 12:107-116.

5. Dunn W: Integrated related services. In: Meyer L, Peck C, & Brown L, eds. *Critical Issues in the Lives of People with Severe Disabilities*. Baltimore, MD: Paul H. Brookes Publishing; 1991; 353-377.

6. Giangreco MF: Delivery of therapeutic services in special education programs for learners with severe handicaps. *Physical & Occupational Therapy in Pediatrics*, 1986;6(2):5-15.

7. Hylton J, Reed P, Hall S, Cicirello N: *The Role of the Physical and Occupational Therapist in the School Setting. (TIES: Therapy in Educational Settings)*. Roseburg, OR: Oregon Department of Education, Regional Services for Students with Orthopedic Impairment; 1987.

8. *Irving Independent School District v. Tatro*, 104 S. Ct. 3371, 1984.

9. Lehr D, Haubrich P: Legal precedents for students with severe handicaps. *Exceptional Children*. 1986;52(4): 358-365.

10. Martin K: Physical therapists in educational environments: Focus on educational significance. *Totline*, 1988;14(2):4.

11. Ottenbacher K: Occupational therapy and special education: Some issues and concerns related to Public Law 94-142. *American Journal of Occupational Therapy*. 1982;36(2),81-84.

12. Osborne AG Jr: How the courts have interpreted the related services mandate. *Exceptional Children*. 1984;51(3) 249-252.

13. Rainforth B, York J: Integrating related services in community instruction. *Journal of the Association for Persons with Severe Handicaps*. 1987;12(3):190-198.

14. Sears C: The transdisciplinary approach: A process of compliance with public law 94-142. *Journal of the Association for Persons with Severe Handicaps*. 1981;6:22-29.

15. Vitello SJ: The Tatro case: Who gets what and why. *Exceptional Children.* 1986;52(4) 353-356.

16. Zirkel PA, Knapp S: Related services for students with disabilities: What educational consultants need to know. *Journal of Educational and Psychological Consultation. 1993;4(2):137-151.*

17. Giangreco MF: Effects of integrated therapy: A pilot study. *Journal of the Association for Persons with Severe Handicaps.* 1986; 11(3):205-208.

18. Giangreco MF: Effects of a consensus-building process on team decision-making: Preliminary data. *Physical Disabilities: Education and Related* Services. 1994;13(1):41-56.

19. Sirvis B: Developing IEPs for physically handicapped students: A transdisciplinary viewpoint. *Teaching Exceptional Children. 1978;10(3):78-82.*

20. Peterson C: Support Services. In: Wilcox B, York R eds. *Quality Education for the Severely Handicapped.* Washington, DC: U.S. Department of Education; 1980; 136-163.

21. Rainforth B, York J, Macdonald C: *Collaborative Teamwork: Integrated Therapy Services in Educational Programs for Students with Severe Disabilities.* Baltimore, MD: Paul H. Brookes;1992.

22. Giangreco MF, Edelman S, Dennis R: Common professional practices that interfere with the integrated delivery of related services. *Remedial and Special Education.* 1991;12(2):16-24.

23. Giangreco MF, Dennis R, Edelman S, Cloninger C: Dressing your IEPs for the educational climate: Analysis of IEP goals and objectives for students with multiple disabilities. *Remedial and Special Education.* 1994; 15(5) 288-296.

24. Bailey DB: A triaxial model of the interdisciplinary team and group process. *Exceptional Children.* 1984;51(1):17-25.

25. Giangreco MF: Making related service decisions for students with severe disabilities: Roles, criteria, and authority. *Journal of The Association for Persons with Severe Handicaps.* 1990;15(1):22-31.

26. Carr SH: Louisiana's criteria of eligibility for occupational therapy services in the public school system. *American Journal of Occupational Therapy.* 1989;43(8):503-508.

27. Effgen SK: Determining school therapy caseloads based upon severity of needs for services. *Totline.* 1984;10(2):16-17.

28. Farley SK, Sarracino T, Howard PM: Development of a treatment rating in schools systems: Service determination through objective measurement. *American Journal of Occupational Therapy.* 1991;45(10):898-906.

29. Hall L, Robertson W & Turner MA: Clinical reasoning process for service provision in the public schools. *American Journal of Occupational Therapy.* 1992;46(10) 927-936.

30. Letters to the Editor: More concerns about Louisiana criteria. *American Journal of Occupational Therapy.* 1990;44(5):470.

31. Giangreco M, Putnam J: Supporting the education of students with severe disabilities in regular education environments. In: Meyer LH, Peck C, Brown L,

eds. *Critical Issues in the Lives of People with Severe Disabilities.* Baltimore, MD: Paul H. Brookes Publishing Co., 1991; 245-270.

32. Giangreco M, Dennis R, Cloninger C, Edelman S, Schattman R: "I've counted Jon": Transformational experiences of teachers educating students with disabilities. *Exceptional Children.* 1993;59(4):359-372.

33. Orelove F, Sobsey R: *Transdisciplinary Approach to Educating Children with Multiple Handicaps.* Baltimore, MD: Paul H. Brookes Publishing; 1987.

34. Giangreco MF, Cloninger C, Mueller P, Yuan S, Ashworth S: Perspectives of parents whose children have dual sensory impairments. *Journal of Association for Persons with Severe Handicaps.* 1991;16(1):14-24.

35. Giangreco MF: Making related service decisions for students with severe handicaps in public schools: Roles, criteria, and authority. *Dissertation Abstracts International.* Dec. 1989;50(6A):1624A. No. DA8919 516.

36. Bowden J, Thorburn J: Including a student with multiple disabilities and visual impairment in her neighborhood school. *Journal of Visual Impairment & Blindness.* 1993;87(7):268-272.

37. Nisbet J, Clark M, Covert S: Living it up! An analysis of research on community living. In: Meyer LH, Peck C, Brown L, eds. *Critical Issues in the Lives of People with Severe Disabilities.* Baltimore, MD: Paul H. Brookes Publishing Co., 1991; 115-144.

38. Sowers J, Hall S, Rainforth B: Related service personnel in supported employment: Roles and training needs. *Rehabilitation Education.* 1990;4:319-331.

39. Dattillo J: Recreation and leisure: A review of the literature and recommendations for future directions. In: Meyer LH, Peck C, Brown L, eds. *Critical Issues in the Lives of People with Severe Disabilities.* Baltimore, MD: Paul H. Brookes Publishing Co., 1991; 171-194.

40. Reichle J, York J, Sigafoos J: *Implementing Augmentative and Alternative Communication: Strategies for Learners with Severe Disabilities* Baltimore, MD: Paul H. Brookes Publishing; 1991.

41. Giangreco MF: *Vermont Interdependent Services Team Approach: A Guide to Coordinating Educational Support Services.* Burlington, VT: University of Vermont, University Affiliated Program of Vermont; 1994.

42. Thousand J, Villa R: Collaborative teams: A powerful tool in school restructuring. In: Villa R, Thousand J, Stainback W, Stainback S, eds. *Restructuring for Caring and Effective Schools: An Administrative Guide to Creating Heterogeneous Schools.* Baltimore, MD: Paul H. Brookes Publishing; 1992; 73-108.

43. Giangreco MF, Cloninger CJ, Iverson V: *Choosing Options and Accommodations for Children: A Guide to Planning Inclusive Education.* Baltimore, MD: Paul H. Brookes Publishing; 1993.

44. Downing J: Active versus passive programming: A critique of IEP objectives for students with the most severe disabilities. *Journal of the Association for Persons with Severe Handicaps.* 1988;13(3):197-201.

45. *Sacramento City Unified School District v. Rachel H.* 14 F3d. 1398, 9th Cir. 1994.

46. Giangreco MF, Baumgart D, Doyle MB: Including students with disabilities in general education classrooms: How it can facilitate teaching and learning. *Intervention in School and Clinic.* in press.

47. Giangreco MF, Eichinger J: Related services and the transdisciplinary approach: A parent/professional training module. In: Anketell M, Bailey EJ, Houghton J, O'Dea A, Utley B, Wickham D, eds. *A Series of Training Modules for Educating Children and Youth with Dual Sensory and Multiple Impairments.* Monmouth, OR: Teaching Research Publications; 1991.

48. Reynolds M: A framework for considering some issues in special education. *Exceptional Children.* 1962;28:367-370.

49. Giangreco M, York J, Rainforth, B: Providing related services to learners with severe handicaps in educational settings: Pursuing the least restrictive option. *Pediatric Physical Therapy.* 1989;1(2):55-63.

50. York J, Rainforth B, Giangreco M: Transdisciplinary teamwork and integrated therapy: Clarifying the misconceptions. *Pediatric Physical Therapy.* 1990;2(2):73-79.

51. Dennis RE, Williams W, Giangreco MF, Cloninger CJ: Quality of life as a context for planning and evaluation of services for people with disabilities. *Exceptional Children.* 1993;59(6):499-512.

52. Giangreco MF, Cloninger CJ, Dennis RE, Edelman SW: National expert validation of COACH: Congruence with exemplary practice and suggestions for improvement. *The Journal of the Association for Persons with Severe Handicaps.* 1993;18(2):109-120.

Assessment and Intervention in School-Based Practice: Answering Questions and Minimizing Discrepancies

Anita C. Bundy

SUMMARY. Assessment and intervention are two of the primary roles of occupational therapists and physical therapists working in public schools. This article conceptualizes a non-linear process of assessment and intervention that maximizes the likelihood that therapists will be integral and valuable members of the educational teams of students with disabilities. An assessment process is described that answers questions about discrepancies between a student's performance and the expectations of others. This is followed by considerations for setting goals and objectives, determining the services to be provided, determining the service delivery setting, and providing intervention that most efficiently and effectively assists students to meet their goals and objectives. *[Article copies available from The Haworth Document Delivery Service: 1-800-342-9678.]*

Occupational therapists (OTs) and physical therapists (PTs) enable students to do what they need and want to do in school. Therapists can assist students with expressing what they have learned, assuming the student

Anita C. Bundy, ScD, OTR/L, FAOTA, is Associate Professor, Department of Occupational Therapy, Colorado State University, 220 OT Building, Fort Collins, CO 80523.

[Haworth co-indexing entry note]: "Assessment and Intervention in School-Based Practice: Answering Questions and Minimizing Discrepancies." Bundy, Anita C. Co-published simultaneously in *Physical & Occupational Therapy in Pediatrics* (The Haworth Press, Inc.) Vol. 15, No. 2, 1995, pp. 69-88; and: *Occupational and Physical Therapy in Educational Environments* (ed: Irene R. McEwen) The Haworth Press, Inc., 1995, pp. 69-88. Single or multiple copies of this article are available from The Haworth Document Delivery Service [1-800-342-9678, 9:00 a.m - 5:00 p.m. (EST)].

role (i.e., behaving in ways expected of students and performing necessary nonacademic tasks, e.g., turning in work on time, getting along with classmates), performing self-care tasks, and improving posture and mobility.[1] Further, because of their unique training, therapists can assist other educational team members to better understand students with special needs, develop more effective strategies for interacting with students, and develop skills necessary for managing students' specialized physical needs (e.g., positioning, feeding).[2]

Clearly, therapists can assume a number of roles within any school setting. However, therapists rarely assume all possible roles for any student. Their roles are determined in response to the goals and objectives specified in a student's educational plan and the expertise of other educational personnel.

When there is no student goal explicitly related to therapeutic areas of expertise (i.e., expressing learning, assuming student role, self-care, and mobility) and no acknowledged need for consultation or staff training, then there is no *educationally relevant* justification for an OT or a PT to provide any service to that student. Eligibility criteria built around individual student objectives are far easier to explain and defend than are criteria based on discrepancies between student's motor skills and their chronological or mental age or the presence of a disabling condition.[1,3]

CONCEPTUALIZING THE INTERVENTION PROCESS

Assessment and intervention are the two primary functions of therapists. Because they must be tailored to the specific needs of each student within each environment, assessment and intervention are complex functions.

Traditionally, therapists have described assessment and intervention as two of three stages of an intervention process (see Figure 1). However, the difficulty with conceptualizing assessment and intervention in such a linear manner is that it makes the therapist (rather than the student, family, or

FIGURE 1. Traditional Conceptualization of Service Planning

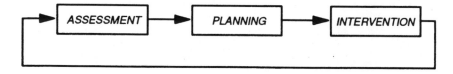

other educational team members) the central figure in a process for making the student more successful at school.

Clearly, the purpose and complex nature of assessment and intervention in educational systems demand a conceptual model that more accurately describes the intervention process. I offer such a model in Figure 2.

In the model shown in Figure 2, I have expanded on the simple 3-step conceptualization by making explicit the tasks in which therapists and other team members engage as they go through the intervention process. As complex as it appears, this model still distorts the process in several important ways. Thus, it must be used with caution.

First, the intervention process, which can be incredibly convoluted, still appears essentially linear. Further, all the numerous educational team members are represented by only two lines. The lower line refers simultaneously to the roles of both the OT and the PT while the upper line refers simultaneously to the roles of all other team members. Not only is this an oversimplification, but separating therapists from other educational team members may also somehow suggest a "we versus they" relationship. That could not be further from my intent; therapists are an integral part of a team. In the sections that follow, I will attempt to capture some of the complexity of the model that cannot be shown in a schematic.

ASSESSMENT: ANSWERING TROUBLESOME QUESTIONS

Assessment is the first stage of the intervention process. As shown in Figure 2, the Assessment Stage consists of a number of parts. Before a therapist is involved, discrepancies between a student's performance and others' expectations become apparent or are anticipated. These discrepancies, in turn, give rise to questions about cause, degree, or ways to minimize or eliminate them. The primary purpose of assessment is to answer those questions.

Selecting an Assessment

Certain types of discrepancies between a student's performance and others' expectations (i.e., assuming the student role, expressing learning, performing self-care or mobility tasks) lead to referrals to OT or PT. The OT or PT, in turn, utilizes any of a number of tools and skills (e.g., interview, observation) to gain insight into the discrepancies. Countless standardized and nonstandardized tests enable PTs and OTs to examine students' skills and any underlying deficits that may explain their difficulties at school.

FIGURE 2. Revised Conceptualization of Service Delivery

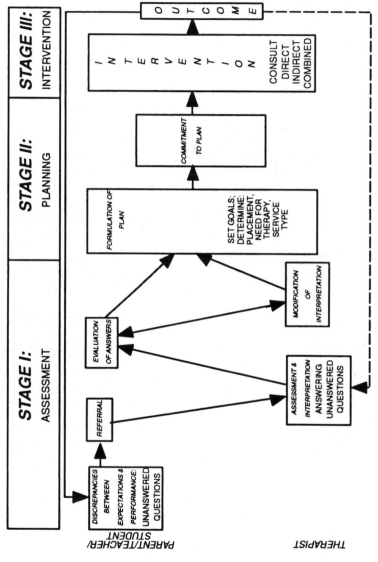

Before using any test, it is important that therapists consider both its purpose and whether it is valid and reliable. If a test has not been demonstrated to have acceptable validity and reliability, we cannot be sure it is measuring what it purports to measure or that a particular student would achieve a similar score on a different day or when evaluated by a different examiner. Thus, considerable caution must be used when reporting results from a test that does not have demonstrated validity and reliability. This advice applies particularly to "homegrown" checklists compiled by therapists in order to examine several areas of concern without spending the time needed to administer multiple standardized tests. If a test is not administered in the standard way, a standard score cannot be derived.

No matter how good the psychometric properties of a test, it is not sensible to administer it unless the results will provide information about the student's difficulties in school. For example, a student whose primary difficulty is handwriting needs to be assessed using tools that will address his or her difficulties with handwriting. After watching a particular student write, preferably in the classroom, the therapist might hypothesize that the student's problems with handwriting are related to underlying sensory integrative dysfunction. Thus, the therapist might administer the Sensory Integration and Praxis Tests (SIPT)[4] to test the hypothesis. Alternatively, the therapist might not administer the SIPT and instead evaluate the student's speed of handwriting and legibility under different environmental conditions. Such an evaluation may or may not yield standard scores. Nevertheless, the information gained by observing through a therapist's trained eye may yield far more readily useable information than would a standardized score.

No substitute exists for observing the student engaged in school activities. Observational assessment enables the therapist to view the student's strengths and difficulties firsthand and adds considerable information about the student's educationally-related needs. In fact, so much information can be gained in this way that the amount of time required for formal assessment can be reduced greatly.

Interview is another powerful assessment tool. Like observation, interview of a student, teacher, and parent yields information that cannot be gathered in any other way. In a half-hour interview, members of the educational team can paint a verbal picture of the student that saves hours of observation and formal assessment time.

Interview also is one of the best ways to learn how the student's difficulties are affecting others' abilities to parent or teach the student. This information is crucial to determining whether consultation is the best way to meet a student's educational needs.

Interpreting and Being Interpreted

Observing, interviewing, and administering formal tests comprise only a part of assessment. If these tools are to be useful, the therapist must interpret their results for other team members. Interpretation involves much more than reporting a score; it means giving meaning to the findings. Thus, assessment is a process by which therapists give other team members access to their profession's theories and to their specialized knowledge about disabling conditions.

As a therapist interprets the results of an assessment, other team members evaluate the adequacy of that assessment and interpretation. Whether they do so consciously or unconsciously, alone or together, these individuals attempt to match what they know about the student with the therapist's descriptions. If the match is good, then the educational team can understand the student's needs or behavior in a new way. If the match is not good, then team members may minimize the potential contributions of therapy toward improving the student's performance in school. Thus, a clear interpretation of the findings is invaluable.

Therapists' knowledge about students can sometimes be tacit. That is, their knowledge is so much a part of them that they find it difficult to articulate. Tacit understanding of a student's difficulties sometimes leads to an incomplete interpretation of assessment findings. Team members, in turn, may receive the interpretation with little enthusiasm. If therapists are sensitive to cues of other team members suggesting that their explanations have "missed the mark," then they can sometimes modify the interpretation to include those things most important to the educational team members. In the following example, the interpretation of the therapist might have been modified, but, unfortunately, was not.

> Stephen is a 6-year-old student in an early childhood special education classroom. Stephen's presenting problems suggested that an evaluation of his sensory integrative function was indicated. The OT, in fact, did find that Stephen had sensory integrative dysfunction; he was dyspraxic (poor motor planning) and demonstrated signs of tactile defensiveness (fight or flight reaction to unexpected or light touch). However, when the OT presented the summary of his findings, he emphasized Stephen's difficulties with balance and gross and fine motor coordination. Stephen's parents and his teacher acknowledged the OT's findings, saying, "He's the expert. If he says Stephen has balance problems, then he probably does, but we don't see them at home. At home Stephen jumps to the very edge of the trampoline, stays there, and then jumps back into the middle. He's in

perfect control. So, if he does have a balance problem, it doesn't seem to get in his way. . . . What we're *really* concerned with is his behavior. Stephen *has to get his behavior under control*. Otherwise, he'll never be able to go to friends' houses and play with the other kids. *Behavior is Stephen's real problem.*"

Unfortunately, Stephen's parents did *not* have this conversation directly with the school OT. . . . Had Stephen's OT inquired . . . about how well the occupational therapy assessment helped to explain Stephen's difficulties in school, he would have given himself the chance to *modify his interpretation*. Because the OT did not ask, he did not have that chance. Further, he failed to convey important information about how occupational therapy could be instrumental in helping Stephen to assume the student role. While Stephen's parents agreed that he should have occupational therapy at school, they did not feel that it was a vital part of his program. The same lack of enthusiasm for occupational therapy was true of Stephen's teacher who also felt that Stephen's problem was primarily behavioral in origin and that what he *really* needed was a good behavior modification program.

By modifying the interpretation, we do not mean that the OT would have changed Stephen's test scores. We mean simply that he would have been able to use his knowledge of sensory integration theory to *expand* his interpretation by explaining Stephen's behavior–his reactions to unexpected touch and noise and his distractibility. Rather than emphasizing his motor incoordination, the therapist could have stressed how sensory integrative dysfunction seemed to be interfering with his ability to behave appropriately in school, at home, and with his friends. In so doing, he probably would have established his services as key to Stephen's educational program, rather than an "extra" service that might, or might not, be very important.[2(p17)]

The notion that others assess the adequacy of our findings and that we can sometimes modify interpretation of our findings is not generally described in therapeutic literature. However, the idea that other team members sometimes disagree with or misunderstand the assessment findings is not new. Once therapists become consciously aware of the processes of other team members, they can seek to elicit more and better information from them. In turn, therapists have the opportunity to improve their interpretations and, ultimately, the quality of their interventions.

In addition to explaining some of the discrepancies between a student's performance and others' expectations, the results of the assessment help to determine whether therapy is warranted. If therapeutic practice models help to explain some of the important discrepancies between expectations and student performance, then the therapist joins with other team members to develop the individualized educational program (IEP). The final decision about whether therapy is educationally relevant for a particular student rests with the team. Therapists cannot make this decision unilaterally.

PLANNING: CREATING THE MAP

With respect to occupational therapy and physical therapy, four important plans emerge from the IEP meeting: (a) a list of carefully-selected goals and educational objectives for the student; (b) specification of the educational placement; (c) determination of the need for occupational therapy and physical therapy; and (d) determination of the most effective types of service delivery.[2]

Setting Goals and Objectives: Selecting the Destination

Of all these IEP outcomes, the most important are the goals and objectives. As the Cheshire Cat commented in *Alice's Adventures in Wonderland,* "If you don't know where you're going, you'll probably never get there." All other decisions hinge on the goals and objectives. In fact, all are simply ways of meeting the goals and objectives.[2,5,6]

As related service providers, OTs and PTs have a responsibility to: (a) familiarize themselves with the educational expectations for the student, (b) collaborate with the team to develop meaningful goals and objectives, and (c) make explicit their potential contributions to the plan. In the best of all situations, the team works together to articulate the most important things a student will know or be able to do differently by the end of the school year. Then one or more team members takes responsibility for each objective.

In some settings, however, each member of the team writes individual objectives that collectively form the IEP. When, out of necessity, OTs and PTs develop recommended objectives independent of other team members, it is their responsibility to complement the teacher's efforts. The relationship between the teacher's objectives and those of the therapist should be explicit.

Far too frequently therapists write objectives that have little obvious relevance to a student's educational needs. Objectives such as: "Jill will hold her head vertically for 5 minutes three times a day," or "Micah will be able to stand on one foot on the balance beam 100% of the time," or "When asked, Billy will maintain the prone extension posture for 30 seconds," should *never* appear on a student's IEP. Aside from the obvious technical difficulties with these objectives (e.g., will Micah have to eat, sleep, and do his math on the balance beam?), they have little apparent relationship to the abilities necessary for these students to succeed in school. Even if . . . a therapist could argue . . . that head control, balance, or extensor muscle tone are underlying abilities that contribute to students' performance of school-related tasks, their relevance is *not obvious* to the members of the educational team. (The school-related task needs to be the objective.) After reading objectives like those for Jill, Micah, and Billy, is it any wonder that teachers and parents often are unsure of the importance of occupational or physical therapy?[2(p21)]

The Setting and the Service

Once a student's objectives are specified, the team determines which program will best enable the student to meet those objectives. PL 94-142 and its successor, the Individuals with Disabilities Education Act (IDEA), clearly state that students should be educated in the least restrictive environment (LRE). As much as possible students with disabilities should be educated with their typically-developing peers. Further, more parents are insisting their children be included in their home schools. Thus, the determination of the LRE is becoming more significant.

OTs and PTs have considerable expertise in adapting environments so that students with disabilities can succeed despite the limitations imposed on them by a disabling condition. Because of their skills for adaptation, PTs and OTs can be instrumental in helping students enter the LRE and helping others in that environment understand and adapt to the needs of the student.

In enabling students to succeed in school, OTs and PTs can deliver service in three different ways: direct service, consultation, and indirect service (monitoring). Frequently, more than one type of service delivery is needed to meet the needs of any particular student.

Each type of service delivery is associated with different types of outcomes and requires different resources. It is the therapist's responsibility to make explicit to the team the anticipated benefits, limitations, and required resources for each type of service delivery as they apply to a specific student. Decisions about types of service delivery rest with the team.

Selecting Consultation

The expected outcome of consultation is that the school environment (human and nonhuman) changes in ways that enable a student to succeed at school despite the limitations imposed by a disabling condition (see Figure 3). Through consultation, parents and teachers can understand a student's behaviors in more positive ways and gain more effective strategies for parenting, teaching, or interacting with the student. In other words, through consultation, parents and teachers become better parents and teachers. Consultation may also result in physical adaptations to classroom materials or facilities in order to allow the student to participate in all aspects of school life.

In consultation, the parent or teacher is the most direct recipient of the therapist's services (see Figure 4). Thus, to consult, the therapist must possess skills for forming a partnership with the consultee and the parent or teacher must see the need for the service. Although consultation can be difficult to administer, it is extraordinarily powerful. In fact, I believe it should be the primary form of service delivery for most students. The reader is referred to other sources[7-13] for additional information.

FIGURE 3. Schematic Representation of Expected Outcomes of Consultation

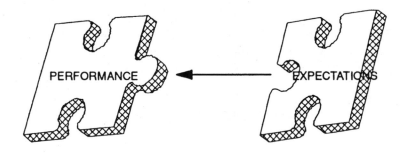

FIGURE 4. Schematic Representation of Consultation

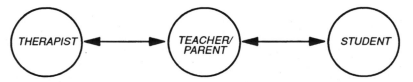

Selecting Indirect Service (Monitoring)

Three outcomes are associated with indirect service. These are: (a) the student refines a skill, (b) the student maintains function, and (c) parents and educators learn to implement a necessary procedure (e.g., positioning, feeding). In indirect service, the therapist teaches a procedure to the teacher, aide, or parent (implementor); the implementor administers the procedure to the student (see Figure 5). Most procedures require fairly sophisticated psychomotor skills. Thus, for indirect service, the therapist must possess good teaching skills.

In addition, because educational personnel are busy, the therapist must have the ability to "sell" the benefits of a particular procedure (especially because classroom aides commonly are the implementors and they often have not been included in the formal planning process). Because of the risks inherent to indirect service (e.g., the possibility of a child's choking during feeding or developing sores because of positioning equipment used incorrectly), it should be used judiciously. More information about providing indirect service is available.[2,9,14]

Selecting Direct Service

In direct service, as with some indirect service, the expected outcome is improved student skill. That is, the student changes in order to meet the expectations of the environment (see Figure 6). In direct service, the student receives "hands on" intervention directly from the PT or OT (see Figure 7). Direct service can be provided in the classroom or in a separate area depending on the needs of the student and the constraints of the classroom.

Although direct service is the type of service delivery most familiar to therapists, it has many limitations. Among the most important of these is the demand on the student's time. A student's need for therapy in school is the result of difficulties keeping up with curricular requirements. Thus, the decision to interrupt the student's participation in school (even in nonacademic activity) should come only when the student needs the skill so badly that the disruption is justified.

FIGURE 5. Schematic Representation of Indirect Service

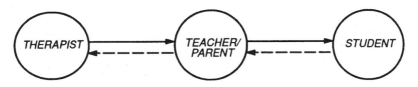

FIGURE 6. Schematic Representation of Expected Outcomes of Direct Service

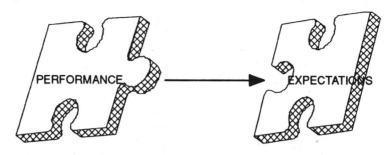

FIGURE 7. Schematic Representation of Direct Service

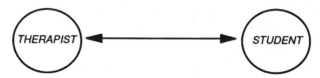

Committing to the Plan

Commitment is defined as "the obligation or pledge to carry out some action or policy or to give support to some policy or person."[15(p457)] Commitment to the plans specified in the IEP is essential. For the therapist, commitment means the team agrees to provide the resources and support necessary for intervention. Commitment comes only when team members understand the educational relevance of the therapist's recommendations and the therapist's recommendations reflect the team's educational concerns for the student.

IMPLEMENTING INTERVENTION: MINIMIZING DISCREPANCIES

Implementation of intervention differs considerably depending on the type of service delivery selected. In the sections that follow, I will describe several important phases of consultation and indirect service (see Figure 8 and 9). For simplicity, I will refer to the consultee as the teacher although parents and aides also assume that role.

FIGURE 8. Phases of Consultation

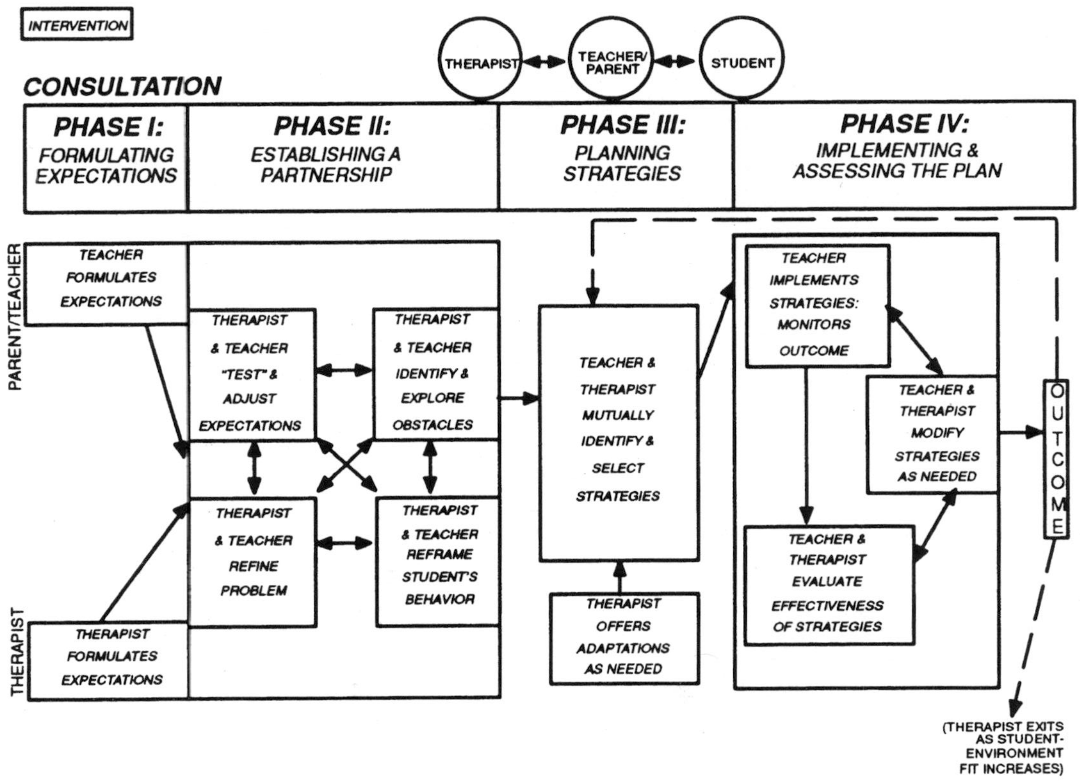

FIGURE 9. Phases of Indirect Service

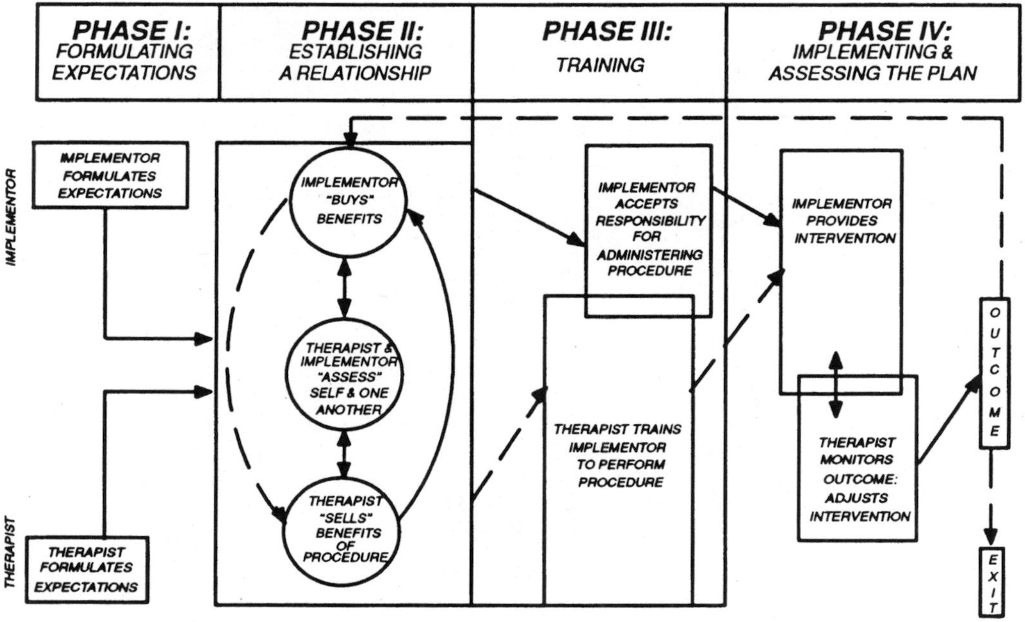

Implementing Consultation

Formulating expectations. Prior to its beginning, both the teacher and the therapist consciously or unconsciously formulate expectations about the intervention process, including what it will be like to work with one another. Although these expectations play an important role in enabling therapists and teachers to prepare for intervention, they are necessarily fiction and must be revised to reflect the real story as it unfolds.[16,17]

Establishing a partnership. Both the teacher and therapist participate as equals in consultation, each contributing his or her skills and unique knowledge of the student. Although the consultative partnership can be difficult to establish, it is the single most important prerequisite to effective collaboration.[2,7,14] To be effective, OTs and PTs must demonstrate their respect for their educator colleagues, be able to share what they know, and be willing to enter into a relationship among equals.

Many things occur during the phase of consultation labelled "Establishing a Partnership" (see Figure 8). They happen in no particular order and rarely are completed before the "Planning Strategies" phase begins.

Knowing that expectations are a part of intervention, the skilled consultant elicits some of the teacher's anticipations and shares his or her own. If necessary, the process of adjusting expectations can begin so that the stories of the two individuals more nearly match.

Refining the problem also is necessary to effective intervention. To refine the problem, the therapist elicits as much information as possible about how the student's difficulties are causing a problem for the teacher in teaching or interacting with the student.

The therapist also uses theories drawn from occupational therapy and physical therapy and knowledge about medical conditions to reframe the problem or an aspect of a student's behavior. The frame through which the teacher views the student's behavior determines how the teacher interacts with the student. Alternative explanations may serve as the basis for formulating more effective teaching strategies.

The therapist also may come to understand the student better by viewing certain aspects of behavior through the teacher's frame of reference. Thus, through consultation, therapists help teachers become better teachers and teachers help therapists become better therapists.

Identifying and exploring obstacles also is an important aspect of consultation. OTs and PTs must remember that the team determined the need for consultation and team members can be important resources. For example, too little time is a commonly-encountered obstacle. If it is not possible to schedule uninterrupted consulting time in any other way, another team member may take periodic responsibility for a classroom to free a teacher.

In a nationwide survey of special education administrators, my colleagues and I[18] asked what one thing therapists could do to improve their effectiveness in schools. These administrators commonly answered, "Be more assertive." Unless consultation teams make their needs known, they will not have them met.

Planning and implementing strategies. New strategies are the primary outcome expected of consultation. These strategies are developed by the teacher and therapist pooling their knowledge and are meant to enable the teacher to teach a particular student in a more effective way. Consultation occasionally includes suggesting adaptive equipment or alternative materials as a means of modifying the environment so that it better fits the needs of a student. It does not include teaching therapeutic procedures. Because strategies developed through consultation are designed to minimize a problem experienced by the teacher and are implemented by the teacher, they must fit the teacher's style, values, and purpose. Only the teacher can determine whether that fit exists.

Implementing Indirect Service (Monitoring)

Establishing a relationship. The therapist/teacher relationship established in indirect service is different in nature and purpose than that of the consultative partnership. Whereas, in consultation, the responsibility for the outcomes is shared, in indirect service, the therapist retains that responsibility. Thus, the relationship between the therapist and the implementor is somewhat hierarchical because the therapist must ensure that the intervention is done properly and without risk to the student. Hierarchical relationships always are difficult to establish and maintain.

Before beginning, the therapist must convince the implementor that the procedure will make a difference in the student's abilities and performance in the classroom. The therapist also must make explicit the expected "costs" of this outcome (e.g., time required to learn and implement the procedure, equipment needed).

Because of the nature of indirect service, the therapist must ask at least two questions before beginning: Is the implementor able to learn the procedure? Am I able to teach the procedure? If therapists cannot administer procedures easily and effectively, then they should not attempt to teach them. Further, if therapists are to teach procedures effectively, they must have access to a variety of teaching strategies.

Implementors also assess their abilities and those of therapists. Unless implementors believe they can learn the procedure and have faith in the therapists' abilities to teach, it is unlikely they will learn the desired skills.

The implementor's assessment of the therapist's ability likely will be based on interactions with that therapist (and with therapists he or she has known previously). He or she may ask, "Does the therapist listen when I talk? Do I feel encouraged or belittled by the therapist? Does the therapist seem genuinely interested in and respectful of me, my opinions, and my job? Will the therapist take time to be sure I have mastered this procedure before I must do it on my own? Will the therapist be available when I encounter difficulties with the procedure?" The more the therapist learns about the implementor's perceptions, the easier it will be to teach the procedure.

Training and implementing the procedure. Training can take place through multiple methodologies (e.g., verbal instruction, observing, practicing), depending on the procedure and the learning style of the implementor. Whatever method is used, the therapist must provide ample time for the implementor to practice and ask questions. Learning occurs through practice.

Even when the implementor appears to have mastered the procedure, the therapist must continue to provide skillful supervision. The therapist does not want to make the implementor feel uneasy, but he or she wants to give the implementor permission to ask questions and request assistance.

Periodically, the therapist assesses the effectiveness of the procedure by evaluating the student's ability to perform the desired skill or by measuring the targeted function. If the development of a particular skill was targeted, the therapist exits when the student has mastered the skill (unless there are other needs). If the purpose of the indirect service was to maintain a function or ability, the therapist's services may be needed for some time. In fact, it may be necessary to train additional personnel to perform the same procedure as the student is promoted from one classroom to another because training should always come directly from a therapist.

Implementing Direct Service

Direct service is the type of service delivery most familiar to therapists, but many questions arise regarding its implementation in schools. The most common of these pertains to the place in which direct service should be administered. Location for direct service is of concern to both therapists and teachers. In fact, Bundy, Lawlor, Kielhofner, and Knecht[18] reported that half of the special education teachers they surveyed *preferred* that direct service be administered outside their classrooms. Bundy concluded that teachers prefer direct service to be conducted outside the classroom when they view it as "a disruption to, rather than an enhancement of, a student's educational program."[2(p15)]

Therapists must be cautious that they actually are facilitating a student's performance of a classroom activity rather than asking the student to attend simultaneously to two unrelated demands as in the following story.

> Mandy was . . . on the floor while her teacher read a story to her and asked questions. The therapist simultaneously . . . facilitate[d postural reactions unnecessary for] the task. . . . Thus, Mandy had to pay attention to the demands of two unrelated tasks, both of which were very difficult for her. The result was that she performed neither very well.[2(p50)]

In order for a student to concentrate intensely on a particular skill, there are times when direct service is best performed outside the classroom. A therapist can design activities that require a student to repeat a particular skill dozens of times rather than doing it only once or twice as often happens when students perform complicated classroom activities that require multiple operations.

One example of the need for direct intervention outside the classroom occurred with Stuart, a second grade student with spastic diplegic cerebral palsy. Stuart climbed stairs so slowly that he missed most of his 15-minute recess period and was often late to class. Climbing stairs more rapidly was one of the objectives in Stuart's IEP. Because the PT was in the building only twice a week, she needed to teach another team member to work on stair climbing with Stuart. Stuart's aide, however, was concerned about his safety and not sure she could learn the skills needed to teach him stair climbing. Thus, the PT spent several short sessions with Stuart, outside the classroom, working on stair climbing and postural reactions. When Stuart was safe, she developed simple procedures for helping his aide work on stair climbing through indirect service.[2]

Direct service *can* be given effectively in the classroom when the therapist works with the student to facilitate the performance of a particular classroom activity *as the activity is occurring*. The benefit to this integrated model of service provision clearly is that students master skills in the contexts in which they normally need them.

CONCLUSION

Practice in schools reflects the essence of occupational therapy and physical therapy for children. OTs and PTs make important and unique contributions to the education of students. By making our reasoning, theories, roles, and services more explicit, we can help others better understand our services.

In this paper, I have described a conceptual model related to assessment and intervention in schools. I described three types of service delivery (direct, indirect, consultation) in terms of the primary recipients of the service delivery and the expected outcomes. I have offered some detail around implementing service although more information is necessary for optimal intervention. Because the focus of consultation is to enable students to succeed despite limitations imposed by a disabling condition, I have argued that consultation should be the primary type of service delivery utilized by OTs and PTs practicing in schools. In general, however, best practice happens when mode of service delivery matches the desired outcome. Thus, combinations of service delivery types are needed to meet the needs of students, teachers, and parents.

REFERENCES

1. Bundy AC. Will I see you in September? The question of educational relevance. *Am J Occup Ther.* 1993;47:848-50.

2. Bundy AC. A conceptual model of practice for school system therapists. In: Bundy AC, ed. *Making a Difference: Occupational and Physical Therapy in Public Schools.* Chicago: University of Illinois at Chicago; 1991.

3. Giangreco MF. More concerns [Letter to the editor]. *Am J Occup Ther.* 1990;44:470.

4. Ayres AJ. *Sensory Integration and Praxis Tests.* Los Angeles, CA: Western Psychological Services; 1989.

5. Bundy AC. *Writing functional goals and objectives.* In: Royeen CB, ed. *AOTA Self Study Series: School-Based Practice for Related Services.* Rockville, MD: American Occupational Therapy Association.

6. Mager RF. *Preparing Instructional Objectives.* Belmont, CA: Fearon; 1975.

7. DeBoer A. *The Art of Consulting.* Chicago, IL: Arcturus Books; 1986.

8. Dunn W. *Pediatric Occupational Therapy.* Thorofare, NJ: Slack; 1990.

9. Chandler BE, Dunn W, Rourk JD. *Guidelines for Occupational Therapy Services in School Systems.* Rockville, MD: American Occupational Therapy Association; 1989.

10. Idol L, Paolucci-Whitcomb P, Nevin A. *Collaborative Consultation.* Austin, TX: Pro-Ed; 1986.

11. Idol L, West JF. Consultation in special education (Part II): training and practice. *J Learn Disab.* 1987;20:474-494.

12. Jaffe EG, Epstein CF. *Occupational Therapy Consultation: Theory, Principles, and Practice.* St. Louis, MO: Mosby; 1992.

13. West JF, Idol L. School consultation (Part I): an interdisciplinary perspective on theory, models, and research. *J Learn Disab.* 1987;20:388-408.

14. Curtin C, Lilly LA, Silber L. When someone else does the intervention: developing effective communication for consultation and indirect service. In:

Bundy AC, ed. *Making a Difference: Occupational and Physical Therapy in Public Schools*. Chicago, IL: University of Illinois at Chicago; 1991.

15. Merriam G, Merriam C. *Webster's Third New International Dictionary* (unabridged). Chicago, IL: Encyclopedia Britannica; 1966.

16. Mattingly CF. *Thinking with Stories: Story and Experience in a Clinical Practice*. Cambridge, MA: Massachusetts Institute of Technology; 1989. Unpublished doctoral dissertation.

17. Mattingly CF, Fleming MH. *Clinical Reasoning: Forms of Inquiry in a Therapeutic Practice*. Philadelphia, PA: FA Davis; 1994.

18. Bundy AC, Lawlor MC, Kielhofner GW, Knecht, HD. Educators' and therapists' perceptions of school system practice. Presented at the annual conference of the American Occupational Therapy Association; June, 1989; Baltimore, MD.

Challenges of Interagency Collaboration: Serving a Young Child with Severe Disabilities

Barrie O'Connor

SUMMARY. Services for young children with severe disabilities typically involve interaction with a wide range of professions and agencies. Although staff members in each agency may have a clear view of their own objectives, it is often the parents who assume responsibility for understanding the complementarity of these services and for coordinating information sharing among them.

This paper explores the nature of interagency cooperation that occurred for one family over a two-year period. Apart from a shared placement in a child care center and a special school which included teachers and therapists, the child also required a range of medical services. The paper critically examines the strengths and weaknesses of interagency communication and the role of the mother in coordinating this information. Implications for service providers are also examined. *[Article copies available from The Haworth Document Delivery Service: 1-800-342-9678.]*

INTRODUCTION

In recent years, the literature on services to children with disabilities has highlighted both the importance of parental involvement on profes-

Barrie O'Connor, PhD, is Senior Lecturer (Human Services), School of Social Sciences, Queensland University of Technology, Beams Road, Carseldine Q 4034, Australia.

[Haworth co-indexing entry note]: "Challenges of Interagency Collaboration: Serving a Young Child with Severe Disabilities." O'Connor, Barrie. Co-published simultaneously in *Physical & Occupational Therapy in Pediatrics* (The Haworth Press, Inc.) Vol. 15, No. 2, 1995, pp. 89-109; and: *Occupational and Physical Therapy in Educational Environments* (ed: Irene R. McEwen) The Haworth Press, Inc., 1995, pp. 89-109. Single or multiple copies of this article are available from The Haworth Document Delivery Service [1-800-342-9678, 9:00 a.m - 5:00 p.m. (EST)].

sional teams and the need for closer collaboration across agencies. Each area is briefly considered as a background to reporting one aspect of a wider research study on interprofessional and interagency teamwork supporting a child with severe disabilities.

The importance of parents as strong advocates and informed consumers of services for their children with disabilities is well established in the literature.[1-4] Turnbull, Blue-Banning, Behr and Kerns[5] noted the key partnership role intended for parents and professionals as an outcome of Public Law 94-142, but argued that research has found that parents typically play a rather passive role in the Individualized Education Program (IEP) process. Subsequent efforts to provide unified education and care programs for very young children with disabilities involved recognition of the child's family as the service recipient rather than the child alone.[6]

Slentz and Bricker[7] challenged the overemphasis on developing and implementing family evaluation instruments,[8] arguing that these might imply that because a child has special needs, the family might also have problems. They suggested that the early intervention professional should be listening to parents and families and gaining their trust so that parents may have more genuine input into evolving programs for their children and be referred, as necessary, to appropriately skilled personnel.

Concerns about interprofessional and interagency cooperation have had a long history. Particular attention has been paid to the need for teamwork among all parties, and this has variously been described as multidisciplinary,[9,10] interdisciplinary[11] and transdisciplinary.[12-14] More recently, collaborative forms of cooperation have been reported.[3,15]

General agreement exists that the collaborative approach includes "working together in a supportive and mutual beneficial relationship."[15(p5)] When applied to teamwork, collaboration defines a particular style that governs the nature of team member interactions. Three elements are immediately apparent: (a) voluntary engagement in the activity, (b) parity among members, and (c) shared decision-making power.

The emphasis on teamwork stems from the varied educational, health, and welfare needs of children with disabilities; those who have severe and profound disabilities have a particular need for ongoing, integrated support services from many different professions. The Queensland Association of Occupational Therapists argued that "no one professional discipline can adequately serve the needs of all disability groups and that the child's functioning cannot be totally compartmentalized."[16(pp3-4)] Their report noted that it is essential for professionals to work collaboratively in teams and to communicate effectively with each other, a view supported by others.[17,18]

Particular attention has been paid to cooperation of therapists and special educators in the development and implementation of integrated therapy programs for children with severe disabilities.[17,19-22] It has been argued that such children should be assessed in, and have programs developed for, functional activities needed in their everyday environments rather than receive therapy for isolated skills in isolated, clinical environments.[23,24]

Services for children with disabilities and their families typically are offered by different agencies (e.g., government, private, voluntary); for diverse social needs (e.g., health, education, welfare); in locations of varying accessibility (e.g., city, rural); under differing funding arrangements (e.g., government, charitable); utilizing differing eligibility criteria (e.g., age, family income, severity or type of disability) and usually with limited financial and human resources.[25] Because many children with disabilities require access to concurrent, multiple services, their parents confront the prospect of finding appropriate and convenient services and often maintain major responsibility for linking and managing information-sharing among such services.[2,4,26,27]

Over recent decades, professionals have faced a range of difficulties in trying to improve collaboration across agency boundaries. First is their lack of knowledge of the goals, structure, and function of other agencies that can lead to misunderstanding, not only for the professionals who work in them, but also for the clients with whom they work.[28,29] Second, agency self-interest involving territorial disputes and competition for funds may cause some staff members to place the needs of their agency ahead of community needs and thus not cooperate in attempts at interagency collaboration.[29]

Third, inadequate communication among executive and field staff members within an agency can exacerbate attempts at interagency cooperation if the promises of cooperation from executives cannot be implemented by field staff.[27-29] Hall[28] recommended that the same person from each agency should attend meetings to ensure continuity of commitment. Fourth, the stereotypes of other professionals and agencies and consequent lack of trust in handing over confidential information[27,29] has meant that some staff members are reluctant to release information across agencies, although such issues can be handled in a trusting and respectful manner with informed consent from the client.[27]

Fifth, potentially useful links may not eventuate unless the practicalities of the interagency relationship are tested in advance of finalizing a cooperative agreement. Hall[28] described one useful process in which weekly meetings to establish interagency protocols alternated with meetings to test their practicalities against a typical case study presented by each agency's representative. The final problem reported is the missing consumer voice in the deliberations. It has been argued that parent and consumer representatives on interagency teams need power and participation equal to that of other team members.[30]

A number of areas worthy of further empirical investigation have been noted. For example, there is a particular need "to identify the minimal attributes of individuals and groups who can function as a team and efficient strategies to achieve this status."[22(p197)] A similar need to clarify team approaches that best help children to benefit from their educational programs was also reported.[31]

Pryzwansky and Noblit criticized the insufficient use of qualitative methodologies in research on teamwork among special education consultants. They claimed that "qualitative case studies have a unique strength in providing a format to understand the dynamics of a situation, linking context, processes, and outcomes."[32(p297)] They also argued that such studies would provide not only rich data for training special education consultants, but also assist in the generation of hypotheses about the consultation process and add to the knowledge base of practitioners and researchers alike. As part of a wider qualitative study on interprofessional teamwork within and across agencies used by one child with severe disabilities,[33] this paper reports the findings related to interagency collaboration between staff members in a special school and those in a long-day child care center, i.e., one operating from 7:30 a.m. to 5:30 p.m.

METHOD

Participants and Settings

Sarah is a sole parent who, together with daughter Catherine (then almost two years old), returned from out of state to her home town, Riverton [pseudonym], a seaboard capital city in eastern Australia, to be closer to her own parents.

At the commencement of the present study, Catherine was three years old. She had previously been diagnosed as having agenesis of the corpus callosum and Riegers syndrome, an anomaly of the anterior segment of the eye. Although the functions of the corpus callosum are not clearly understood, agenesis usually results in mental retardation, seizures, and motor disturbances.[34] Because Riegers syndrome is often associated with glaucoma, regular checks for this possible complication were needed. Myopia was also found. Catherine displayed significant developmental delays in cognitive, language, social, and motor areas of functioning. She also experienced intermittent and, on occasion, severe seizures in spite of ongoing medication adjustments to manage this condition. She was totally dependent on adults for most of her self-help skills such as eating, toileting, washing, speaking and mobility. She could move from the lying to sitting position only with assistance, but was able to hold her bottle for drinking while lying down.

Figure 1 reveals the agencies with which Catherine and Sarah interacted during their years in Riverton. Such agencies comprised the child care and special school settings in which the study was conducted over a two-year period; respite and after-school nanny care; and medical practitioner and hospital services.

Special School

Sarah wanted more intervention than the infrequent home visits from therapists employed by the government intellectual disability services agency. Soon after Catherine's second birthday, Sarah gained for her a part-time place for three mornings a week at the Riverton Special School. This gave Catherine potential access to more regular occupational, speech, and physical therapy services in an educational context. The teacher and two aides provided educational programs to the six children in Catherine's

FIGURE 1. Interrelationships of Agencies Serving a Child with Severe Disabilities

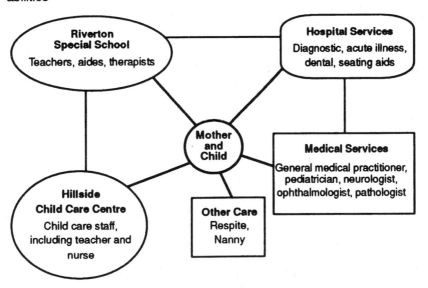

class, both individually and in small groups, along with therapy support. Catherine's attendance was gradually increased to three, and occasionally four, full days a week (9 a.m. to 3 p.m.) towards the end of the school year.

Riverton Special School, a purpose-built government school for those with severe and profound disabilities, had approximately 55 students up to 18 years of age, in 10 classes each with five or six students. Catherine's class was the youngest group in the school. Two part-time physical therapists and two part-time occupational therapists, together with an itinerant speech therapist attending the school one day per week, provided services described as mainly transdisciplinary or consultative in nature.

Child Care

At the beginning of the following year, Sarah returned to full time study and thus required a five day per week placement for Catherine, now three years of age. She also believed that Catherine needed to experience a regular educational environment in which she was surrounded by the stimuli of able-bodied peer models, a belief supported by the special school staff members. Although Catherine was the youngest member of her school class, she was considered the highest functioning. Staff members readily acknowledged the social differences in their own setting of children with profound disabilities who were totally dependent on adults for mobility, communication and other self-help skills. Sarah's aspirations for Catherine's general child care placement were also consonant with the philosophies and practices of integration articulated both by professional and government policies.[35]

Catherine commenced her placement in long-day child care at the Hillside Children's Center in Riverton in January 1989, attending on Mondays and Tuesdays, and continued at the special school for the remaining three days of the week. Hillside was a multifunctional center offering varied early childhood services including kindergarten/preschool, long-day child care, and parent and toddler groups. Long-day child care operated from 7:30 a.m. to 5:30 p.m. week days for all but two weeks in the end-of-year holiday period. Three groups attended: six babies, 12 toddlers under three years of age, and 22 children aged 3 to 5 years. Each group was staffed by two caregivers. Staff member qualifications included child care, teaching, and nursing credentials.

Other Agencies

As the study progressed, it was possible to include, at Sarah's invitation, an examination of additional professional support that Catherine and her mother received. Medical services were provided by a general medical practitioner, pediatrician, neurophysician, ophthalmologist, pedodontist, radiologist and pathologist, together with brief hospitalization periods for vision checks and management of acute seizures. Once Sarah commenced employment, she used both respite care services, usually an overnight stay twice each month, and a nanny for Catherine's after-school care and for those days when Catherine was too ill to attend her regular placements.

The study, which commenced with Catherine's admission to child care in January 1989, followed her access to services for two calendar years, until she and her mother moved to another state in January 1991.

Procedures

A qualitative approach was used, based on the assumption that a rich description and subsequent analysis of the lived experiences of the participants would provide a basis for understanding how interprofessional teamwork and interagency collaboration actually functioned. Grounded theory methodology[36-38] was adopted to guide data collection, data analysis, and theory formulation.

Methods of data collection in qualitative research are not rigidly controlled as in experimental research; some flexibility is needed in recognizing and seizing upon opportunities to collect data that may enrich the pool of information from which theoretical propositions can be made and tested. Although the present study began with a clear focus on the child care and special school settings and the relationships between them, Sarah subsequently suggested that the involvement of the medical practitioners, respite care, and after-school nanny services might also be included in the study.

Data were gathered through direct participant-observation, aided by field notes, audiotaping and videotaping segments of activity in each setting, and through multiple interviews of key participants. Interactions of staff members in meetings, with parents, and in visits to and from other agency professionals were also observed and recorded. Additional documentary information was drawn from attendance records, the child's files, and participant diaries. Research memos were created regularly to reflect on methodological and content concerns. Such qualitative procedures were compatible with those recommended in the literature.[38-41]

OUTCOMES

Several findings arose from the study which have implications not only for interagency collaboration but also for the role of parents in fostering that process. As already noted, widespread agreement exists in the literature that closer collaboration among professionals from different disciplines and agencies can enhance the quality of services offered to children with disabilities and their families. The present study found that an assertive parent advocate can foster closer links among professionals, that professional staff members can create a genuine partnership with parents, that flexible management procedures can enhance interagency cooperation, and that interagency visits lead to a better understanding of complementary efforts. But it also revealed that a more meaningful and integrated therapy and education program might have been achieved had closer organizational links been developed. Each finding is discussed in turn.

Parent as Child's Advocate

Sarah repeatedly took the view that professionals first had to "get to know" her daughter before they commenced any form of intervention with her. She argued that as Catherine's mother, she knew her moods and behaviors best and could interpret the nature of Catherine's responses (e.g., her likes and dislikes) to various professional inputs.

Prior to her arrival in Riverton, Sarah was highly critical of the therapists from one agency who visited for an hour every two weeks and proceeded to manipulate Catherine without first establishing rapport. Sarah recalled, "They didn't get to know Catherine as a friend . . . if they spent more time and became my friend rather than . . . [an] instructor type, that would have alleviated my stress."

In contrast, the occupational therapist she first met at the Riverton Special School took a close interest in Sarah's views of Catherine and sought to build a program based on relevance to the family setting. Similarly, at the child care center staff members first invited Sarah and Catherine for a visit to assess the appropriateness of their program for Catherine's needs. By getting to know her in the setting, and by helping Sarah to become familiar with their routines, they were able to fashion an appropriate placement.

Parent in Partnership with Professionals

Sarah recognized the sense of foreboding in the minds of some child care staff members who were inexperienced in working with children with disabilities. She and the child care center director negotiated a joint meeting between the child care staff members and the special school teacher and occupational therapist who had taught Catherine. Together they explored the potential for interagency collaboration.

As was the case with any other parent helping children to settle by scaffolding a growing relationship between them and the child care staff members, Sarah spent substantial periods in the early weeks of Catherine's child care placement helping the staff get to know her particular ways of communicating and her preferences for feeding and general handling. Sarah was aware of their concerns about Catherine's possible seizures but was also concerned herself about how safely Catherine might be accommodated among a group of highly mobile and at times unsteady toddlers. The latter concern was addressed by Sarah's purchase of a small chair that offered some protection for Catherine. The concern regarding seizures dissipated with the passage of time; only one mild seizure occurred during Catherine's two-year placement in child care, despite the fact that she had experienced frequent seizures at home and on occasions had been hospitalized for acute episodes.

The Hillside staff members consciously chose to develop a partnership relationship[1] with Sarah characterized by effective interpersonal skills of openness and self disclosure, sharing information, showing empathy, problem solving together, and being trusting and trustworthy. The relationship led to sharing concerns such as Catherine's safety, her seizures, her level of inclusion in activities, and staff feelings of guilt about not doing enough to support and foster Catherine's interactions with other children. Neither the parent nor the staff members needed to feel unduly defensive when both the positive and negative aspects of Catherine's inclusion were discussed openly and honestly. They shared responsibility by exchanging expertise and respective perceptions of Catherine's needs and progress, and by jointly owning the problems and the solutions. Staff members did not expect more time and effort than Sarah was able to give. Though their relative efforts were complementary, there was equal respect for each partner in the collaborative relationship.

Flexible Management

Flexibility was found to be as significant in relationships between agencies, as it was in interprofessional teamwork.[33] In the interagency context, flexibility has been defined as "the extent to which agencies are free from formal rules or guidelines that inhibit the services to eligible clients."[27(p187)] The present study supports this view.

Separately, each agency undertook Catherine's placement as an innovative response to a gap in existing services. The challenge for the special school was to place a child several years younger than existing rules allowed and, for the child care center, to enroll a child with severe disabilities for the first time. Personnel at both centers were prepared to examine

Sarah's and Catherine's needs and to respond creatively within the scope of the available resources. Each had places available, but some of the rules had to be changed. Those responsible for making decisions in each center were prepared to challenge existing limits and break new ground in their efforts to accommodate Catherine's enrollment because they believed in the value of their services for her. They judged the balance between costs and benefits to favor Catherine's inclusion.

Elder[27] cautioned against rigid, mechanical adherence to rules that denies the use of rational judgment by agency staff members. Although policy guidelines are needed to facilitate agency activities, effective teamwork can be shackled by inflexible interpretations of such guidelines. The actions of personnel in this study reflected the recommended approach.

Interagency Visits

At the initial meeting of child care and special school staff members, it was agreed that further interaction should occur between staff members from the two centers. The child care staff visited the special school on eight occasions, and reverse visits occurred on four occasions. During these visits, staff members familiarized themselves with programs and activities in the other place and sometimes brought Catherine's peers from each setting for a visit. Most of the visits to the special school were undertaken by new child care staff members to familiarize themselves with Catherine's routines, and on one occasion the toddler group leader attended Catherine's IEP review meeting.

The reciprocal social visits of children and staff members enabled children from each setting to experience each other's company, learning environment, and equipment. Information was gleaned on strategies for handling Catherine and activities that she enjoyed. Much of the discussion related to Catherine's routines in eating, drinking, administration of medication, toileting, communication, sitting, standing, and walking. These routines continued to be the focus of other familiarization visits made to the special school by successive new staff members at Hillside over the two years of the study.

Although such visits increased the general understanding each center's personnel had of the other's programs, staff members were unable to achieve a close, consistent, and genuinely collaborative relationship. Several reasons are offered later in the paper.

Potential for Integrated Programs

The child care staff soon recognized that, although Catherine was suitably placed among a group of toddlers, she was unable to move herself independently and thus could not choose among the range of activities available to her more mobile peers. This meant that staff members had to be constantly on the lookout to include her in activities, by picking her up and moving her from one place to another. They often felt guilty at the end of a day if they believed they had not assisted Catherine as frequently as might be desired to give her as wide a range of choices as her peers enjoyed. An often stated concern in these early months was their desire to seek advice from the special school therapists in helping Catherine to become more independently mobile.

This request was neither easily communicated nor translated into timely action. After the initial meeting, there were only two follow-up visits to the child care center by therapists during Catherine's two years of placement there. Here was a center with a wealth of demands and challenges for daily activity in a regular placement among non-disabled peers, but access to an integrated therapy program was not achieved. Several difficulties, though not insurmountable, were identified.

Barriers to Collaboration

Some major difficulties arose in the demanding day-to-day operations of both the child care center and the special school. In addition, the medical services were found to be insular in their communication networks. Such findings helped to explain why the parent was viewed as a major conduit for incidental communication. Each problem is briefly discussed and the final section suggests ways of resolving such concerns.

Discontinuity in Interagency Communication

The continuity of formal communication between settings was impeded in several ways. First, there were different special school staff members present at the first two visits so that additional time was needed to establish an open and trusting relationship. The participants needed to get to know each other, to explore the nature of their respective programs and to learn how Catherine operated in each setting. In essence, there was a new team forming[42] and some of the expectations raised at the original meeting, such as therapy input at Hillside, were not clarified at the second meeting because there was no therapist present at the point when follow-up action was discussed. The early promise of an occupational therapist follow-up visit to child care did not occur because the therapist transferred soon after to another city. Thus a hiatus occurred in which the therapy support that Hillside staff anticipated did not eventuate until the following October, a delay of ten months.

Second, there were other staff changes over the two years, particularly high in the child care unit, which meant that much of the effort was directed at re-establishing contacts to build the interagency connection. Third, staff members from each center had significant difficulties in contacting each other because of heavy demands made on them during work time, the varying lengths of their respective working days, and even their different holiday breaks. It has been noted that ineffective communication protocols can hinder interagency collaboration.[27-29] In the present study, personnel from both centers appeared unable to arrange time to devote to the shared initiative which, although desirable, in effect became an unexpected additional responsibility.

Fourth, the special school therapists, all employed part-time, did not have time available to meet the wide ranging demands on their services. The physical therapist and the occupational therapist were regularly involved in accompanying children to specialist seating and orthoses clinics at both the hospital and the cerebral palsy center in Riverton, and they valued the professional growth that occurred through such contact with their colleagues in specialist agencies. This activity, however, involved costly staff time for a small number of children each week, and it meant that the majority of children were not seen very frequently in their classroom settings. In addition, therapists were frustrated by excessive delays, not only in gaining appointments for children to be measured for specialist seating, wheelchairs, standing frames and callipers, but also for the subsequent delivery of these items which sometimes arrived so late that they no longer suited the children.

Finally, children's ill health caused the postponement of planned visits by children and staff members between centers on several occasions. These were unpredictable but nonetheless significant events that influenced the course and frequency of interagency contacts.

Professional and Agency Boundaries

Sarah and some special school staff members took the view that the child care personnel might feel overwhelmed at the outset if they thought they would be required on a regular basis to undertake any therapy activities with Catherine at Hillside. Child care staff members already faced heavy demands from very active and mobile children and had little time for programmed one-to-one contact with children. Although individualized contact was highly valued, it occurred only intermittently and spontaneously across the day.

The understanding that child care staff members would not need to be involved in Catherine's therapy program was promoted and appeared to be a "selling point" to secure Catherine's Hillside placement, a view later confirmed by several informants. In addition, the special school therapists were not funded to serve children beyond the school premises, so that any visits to Hillside needed to be negotiated as a special case with the special school principal. The combined effect was to reduce the perceived importance of any therapy input at Hillside. Several concerns arose from this situation.

First, the promise not to overload Hillside staff members may have been partially interpreted by them as needing to respect others' professional and agency boundaries—that they should not become involved in a technical area that was not only beyond their own expertise but also the preserve of a specialist agency. In their visits to the special school, the child care staff members acknowledged their responsibility not to delve into the "therapy aspects" of Catherine's program, perceiving that to be divorced from an integrated IEP. That the therapists maintained their own files separately from each child's IEP file may have reinforced that view. No offer was made by the therapists to integrate their objectives into Catherine's child care program.

Second, there were difficulties that flowed from the informal sharing of information as Hillside personnel visited the special school to understand better Catherine's program and how it might be extended in child care. At one visit a child care staff member observed a new way of walking Catherine that had not been checked with the physical therapist. The visitor later demonstrated it to other child care staff members who mentioned it also to Sarah. The physical therapist later explained:

> Sometimes you have to try things, see how they go, because you think they could work but then once you've done it you realize that it's not going to work and it's totally inappropriate. So for someone to come in and see something like that, some therapy-based program and then take it away and relay it, . . . that's where the danger comes in. Not having therapy-based personnel at Hillside.

Third, while it was agreed that both centers had different goals for Catherine based on the respective strengths of their programs, it seemed that greater integration of this effort could have worked to Catherine's advantage. Certainly Hillside staff members did not have the resources to run concentrated therapy programs each day, but a clearer understanding of therapy goals and close monitoring of appropriate handling techniques by the therapists would have provided greater consistency in Catherine's daily routines. Although the special school had the advantages of specialist therapy and equipment resources, Hillside was able to provide a wide range of meaningful, age-appropriate activities into which Catherine's therapy programs could have been channelled. Here were clear opportunities for an integrated therapy program, had the special school therapists been willing to visit Hillside for regular monitoring sessions. As this was an unusual case in which a special school student enjoyed a shared placement with another community agency, it was disappointing that the restriction on providing services beyond the school was not challenged by any of the participants. Shortcomings of related (therapy) services that are delivered in relative isolation from children's educational programs have been reported[20] while favorable outcomes for therapy programs that have been integrated closely into the total educational programs for children with severe disabilities have also been noted.[31,43]

Fourth, in the first year Hillside staff members had repeatedly, though indirectly, sought therapy advice on giving Catherine some mobility, to enable her to participate more meaningfully in their program. Although their request for a walking aid may have been unacceptable in therapy terms, there was no direct communication to secure alternative solutions or to modify program goals. Without the benefit of close liaison, the Hillside personnel continued to view mobility with assistance as an important short term educational goal while the therapy staff viewed sitting and later standing posture as primary concerns.

Finally, it was not until a formal interagency meeting was held after work one evening in mid-October (10th month of the placement) without Catherine present that the first direct (occupational) therapy advice was given to Hillside staff members in the child care setting. The next visit to Hillside by both the physical therapist and the occupational therapist occurred when Catherine was in attendance, in the 15th month of her 23 month placement there, an opportunity they took to review her seating and her standing frame arrangements and to discover first hand more about Catherine's activities in that setting.

Undemanding Links; Unclear Goals

A comfortable but perhaps insufficiently challenging relationship had emerged between the two centers. In large measure, this may be attributed to the time and personnel resource difficulties already noted. Stability in team membership was necessary for the relationship to mature.

An agreement on common goals they might undertake jointly for Catherine was needed, but this point was not reached. Each agency had different goals for her because they were providing different services. Each center operated within different social contexts and used quite different teaching strategies. Although there was generous and open sharing about aspects of Catherine's behavior and routines at each visit, and the ongoing encounters took place with much goodwill, there were obvious difficulties with follow-through.

Beyond their individualized goals for Catherine, caregivers needed to formalize clear goals for the interagency relationship—those which address the routines of regular contact, responsibility for follow-through, and identification of the strengths and opportunities each can offer the other in the interests of the child and parent. Although the interagency links arose as an avenue of potential support to the child care center staff members, they were more benignly accepted than actively sought.

Parent as Medical Information Conduit

The medical practitioners typically concentrated their communication among themselves, but they indicated a willingness to communicate more widely with teachers and others on request and within the protocols of confidentiality. A general concern remains, however, about the availability and relevance of some medical information provided to practitioners in child care and education, particularly in cases such as Catherine's where much of her learning potential is inextricably linked to her medical impairments. Her condition, agenesis of the corpus callosum, was not fully understood because of its varying effects; thus a clear prognosis was not available to guide ongoing educational programming. Her epilepsy appeared resistant to medical management and her quality of vision remained largely unknown.

In the present study, transmission of such information occurred solely through the parent as interpreter of information from the medical practitioners. This raises the concern that communication distortion may unwittingly occur not only from doctor to parent, but again from parent to teacher or therapist, with consequent implications for the adequacy and safety of programs.

In summary, the difficulties described here need to be seen in a wider, positive, developmental context. The special school had already made a flexible response to Sarah's request that Catherine be admitted to school as a two-year-old. In addition, the Hillside staff members took on the enrollment of a child with severe disabilities for the first time. They did so with the knowledge that the special school would lend support where it could. Personnel at both centers also contributed some of their personal time to ensure that communication could take place after work hours. Such experiences confirm one of Benson's claims for quality work undertaken in interagency coordination—the flexibility in relationships so that interagency personnel can be adaptable in their decisions about client services, rather than be bound by a complex set of rules.[27]

IMPLICATIONS

Several implications for future practices in interagency collaboration have been identified and these are briefly discussed.

Parent as Pivotal Information Transmitter

The study graphically revealed the wide scope of professional and agency contacts that the parent made in gaining access to needed services in medicine, child care, and education. Apart from medical and therapy referrals to specific points of service, the parent acted primarily as a self-advocate in her search for services. In addition, the parent also appeared to be a key pivot in the communication from one agency to another, either encouraging greater direct communication between agency staff members, or else carrying and sharing the information herself as she moved between locations. The effects, both on parents and on the accuracy of information relayed to others, need further investigation.

A central question remains: Is there any medical information held by doctors that might be useful to child care and education professionals or to therapists that could profitably be communicated more directly to these professionals, with the appropriate permission from parents? Although it may be argued that parents have sole right to determine how information about their children is shared among agencies, not all families would necessarily have the skills and insights to handle this effectively. Medical practitioners often hold information that is important in the development of educational programs, particularly for children with severe disabilities, but either may not be aware of its relevance and thus do not pass it on to parents and other relevant professionals, or such information may be distorted in its transmission.

A British report[44] has highlighted the need for a balanced partnership that empowers parents to gain control and understanding of decisions affecting their child, in contrast to the power relationships inherent in a professional expert model[1,45] in which patients are only told what doctors feel they should hear or in which physicians withhold information in the belief that patients would ask questions if they wanted answers or that they would find too much information upsetting.

Similarly, teachers and therapists may not ask for such information and thus overlook its importance in program planning. Perhaps the usual practice of restricting communication mainly within one's own professional channels needs to be challenged. Further research is needed in this area.

Strengthening Links Between the Agencies

The major part of the interagency focus of this study was the relationship between the child care center and the special school. Although staff members at each place sought to engage in a genuinely collaborative effort, there were obvious shortcomings mostly beyond their control. Yet, current realities are open to challenge and change, and solutions need to be sought for the difficulties found. Several possibilities are suggested as challenges to be faced.

Building Trust in Interagency Teamwork

It has been noted that for "professionals to interact with each other in a truly collaborative manner, the elements of trust, respect, and mutual dependence must be present."[46(p17)] Hall also emphasized the importance of "mutual trust, openness, clarity and compromise"[28(p53)] by injecting what he termed the "human factor" into interagency cooperation. The human factor was clearly evident in the way in which staff related to children and parents in both centers. Professionals who understand and practice interpersonal skills, such as genuineness, empathy, trust, respect, openness, problem solving, assertion, and confrontation, enhance their relationships with colleagues and their clients. It is argued that these professionals have the cognitive and affective scaffolding that affords richer insight into interprofessional and interagency collaboration.

Identifying Common Goals

Another challenge emerging from this study is the need to set clear goals for interagency collaboration. Although the relationships between agencies might be valued for their informality, more effectively integrated programs could be developed for the client if common goals are identified. The benefits to teamwork derived from the synergy of members' interdependent efforts,[47] can also be translated into the arena of interagency collaboration. Utilizing the respective strengths of each agency's resources in a flexible manner can create service opportunities not easily achieved by either agency operating alone.

Focusing Interagency Management

Effective teams require consistent and appropriate membership, comprised of people with skills to contribute to team goals.[47] Where there is a high turnover in staff, there is consequent discontinuity in interagency contact and the need for time to rebuild interagency teams.

Given that staff turnover is a reality and access to meeting times for a large group of interagency personnel is difficult, interagency cooperation may be best organized and monitored by a small group of professionals whose membership is stable–perhaps just one from each agency–and whose goals are clearly focused on strategic management of the collaborative effort.

CONCLUSION

The present study indicates that effective links between agencies may be compromised by discontinuity in interagency communication, by perceived professional boundaries, by unrealistic demands placed on parents as communicators of key data, and by unclear goals for collaboration. The findings challenge professionals to adopt a collaborative approach with each other and with parents, and to improve interagency links by building trust, by setting common goals, by creating an interagency management team with a focused and stable membership, and by valuing flexibility in their agency relationships.

AUTHOR NOTE

The author acknowledges John Elkins for his helpful advice and reflection on the wider study from which this paper was drawn.

REFERENCES

1. Cunningham C, Davis H. *Working with Parents: Frameworks for Collaboration*. Milton Keynes, England: Open University Press; 1985.

2. Gorham KA. A lost generation of parents. *Exceptional Children*. 1975;41:521-524.

3. Rainforth B, York J, Macdonald C. *Collaborative Teams for Students with Severe Disabilities: Integrating Therapy and Educational Services*. Baltimore, MD: Paul H. Brookes; 1992.

4. Turnbull AP, Turnbull HR. *Families, Professionals and Exceptionalities*. Columbus, OH: Charles E. Merrill; 1986.

5. Turnbull AP, Blue-Banning M, Behr S, Kerns G. Family research and intervention: a values and ethical examination. In: Dozecki PR, Zaner RM, eds. *Eth-*

ics of Dealing with Persons with Severe Handicaps: Towards a Research Agenda. Baltimore, MD: Paul H. Brookes; 1986: 119-140.

6. Krauss MW. New precedent in family policy: individualized family service plan. *Exceptional Children.* 1990;56:388-395.

7. Slentz KL, Bricker D. Family-guided assessment for IFSP development: jumping off the family assessment bandwagon. *Journal of Early Intervention.* 1992;16:11-19.

8. Bailey DB Jr, Simeonsson RJ. Assessing needs of families with handicapped infants. *The Journal of Special Education.* 1988;22:117-127.

9. Andrews RJ. Multi-disciplinary models in special education? *The Slow Learning Child.* 1975:22:45-57.

10. Bardon JI. Viewpoints on multidisciplinary teams in schools. *School Psychology Review.* 1983;12:186-189.

11. Holm VA, McCartin RE. Interdisciplinary child development team: team issues and training in interdisciplinariness. In: Allen KE, Holm VA, Schiefelbusch RL, eds. *Early Intervention: A Team Approach.* Baltimore, MD: University Park Press; 1978: 97-122.

12. Baine D, Sobsey R, McDonald L. Transdisciplinary decision-making. *Canadian Journal of Special Education.* 1987;3:79-87.

13. Magrun WM, Tigges KN. A transdisciplinary mobile intervention program for rural areas. *Am J Occup Ther.* 1982;36:90-94.

14. York J, Rainforth B, Giangreco MF. Transdisciplinary teamwork and integrated therapy: clarifying the misconceptions. *Pediatr Phys Ther.* 1990;2:73-79.

15. Friend M, Cook L. *Interactions: Collaboration Skills for School Professionals.* New York, NY: Longmans; 1992.

16. The Queensland Association of Occupational Therapists. *Standards of Professional Practice for Occupational Therapists Working in Paediatrics.* Unpublished manuscript. Author; 1986, June.

17. Giangreco MF, York J, Rainforth B. Providing related services to learners with severe handicaps in educational settings: pursuing the least restrictive option. *Pediatr Phys Ther.* 1989;1:55-63.

18. Sparling JW. The transdisciplinary approach with the developmentally delayed child. *Phys Occup Ther Pediatr.* 1980;1(2):3-15.

19. Campbell PH. The integrated programming team: an approach for coordinating professionals of various disciplines in programs for students with severe multiple handicaps. *Journal of The Association for Persons with Severe Handicaps.* 1987;12:107-116.

20. Giangreco MF, Edelman S, Dennis R. Common professional practices that interfere with the integrated delivery of related services. *Remedial and Special Education.* 1991;12(2):16-24.

21. Lyon S, Lyon G. Team functioning and staff development: a role release approach to providing integrated educational services for severely handicapped students. *Journal of The Association for Persons with Severe Handicaps.* 1980;5:250-263.

22. Rainforth B, York J. Integrating related services in community instruction. *Journal of The Association for Persons with Severe Handicaps.* 1987;12:190-198.

23. Downing J, Bailey BR. Sharing the responsibility: using a transdisciplinary team approach to enhance the learning of students with severe disabilities. *Journal of Educational and Psychological Consultation.* 1990;1:259-278.

24. Sternat J, Messina R, Nietupski J, Lyon S, Brown L. Occupational and physical therapy services for severely handicapped students: toward a naturalized public school service delivery model. In: Sontag E, Smith J, Certo N, eds. *Educational Programming for the Severely and Profoundly Handicapped.* Reston, VA: Division of Mental Retardation, The Council for Exceptional Children; 1977: 263-266.

25. Audette RH. Interagency collaboration: the bottom line. In: Elder JO, Magrab PR, eds. *Coordinating Services to Handicapped Children: A Handbook for Interagency Cooperation.* Baltimore, MD: Paul H. Brookes; 1980: 25-34.

26. Brotherson MJ, Goldstein BL. Time as a resource and constraint for parents of young children with disabilities: implications for early intervention services. *Topics in Early Childhood Special Education.* 1992;12:508-527.

27. Elder JO. Essential components in development of interagency collaboration. In: Elder JO, Magrab PR, eds. *Coordinating Services to Handicapped Children: A Handbook for Interagency Cooperation.* Baltimore, MD: Paul H. Brookes; 1980: 181-201.

28. Hall HB. The intangible human factor: the most critical coordination variable. In: Elder JO, Magrab PR, eds. *Coordinating Services to Handicapped Children: A Handbook for Interagency Cooperation.* Baltimore, MD: Paul H. Brookes; 1980: 45-62.

29. Kramer RM. Dynamics of teamwork in the agency, community, and neighborhood. *Social Work.* 1956;1(1):56-62.

30. Everson JM, Moon MS. Transition services for young adults with severe disabilities: defining professional and parental roles and responsibilities. *Journal of The Association for Persons with Severe Handicaps.* 1987;12:87-95.

31. Giangreco M. Effects of integrated therapy: a pilot study. *Journal of The Association for Persons with Severe Handicaps.* 1986;11:205-208.

32. Pryzwansky WB, Noblit GW. Understanding and improving consultation practice: the qualitative case study approach. *Journal of Educational and Psychological Consultation.* 1990;1:293-307.

33. O'Connor BA. *Interprofessional Teamwork and Interagency Collaboration Supporting a Young Child with Severe Disabilities.* Unpublished doctoral dissertation, The University of Queensland, St Lucia, Australia; 1994.

34. Ritter S. Educational intervention with a primary school girl with agenesis of the corpus callosum. *The Exceptional Child.* 1981;28:65-72.

35. Australian Early Childhood Association. *Integrating Children with Disabilities into Child Care Services: Using Supplementary Service Grants.* Watson, ACT, Australia: Author; 1988.

36. Glaser BG, Strauss, AL. *The Discovery of Grounded Theory: Strategies for Qualitative Research.* London, England: Weidengold & Nicolson; 1968.

37. Strauss AS. *Qualitative Analysis for Social Scientists*. Cambridge, England: Cambridge University Press; 1987.

38. Strauss A, Corbin J. *The Basics of Qualitative Research: Grounded Theory Procedures and Techniques*. Newbury Park, CA: Sage; 1990.

39. Spradley JP. *The Ethnographic Interview*. New York, NY: Holt, Rinehart and Winston; 1979.

40. Spradley JP. *Participant Observation*. New York, NY: Holt, Rinehart and Winston; 1980.

41. Stainback SB, Stainback WC. *Understanding and Conducting Qualitative Research*. Dubuque, IA: Kendall/Hunt; 1988.

42. Kormanski C, Mozenter A. A new model of team building: a technology for today and tomorrow. In: Pfeiffer JW, ed. *The 1987 Annual: Developing Human Resources*. San Diego, CA: University Associates; 1987: 255-267.

43. Campbell PH, McInerney WF, Cooper MA. Therapeutic programming for students with severe handicaps. *Am J Occup Ther.* 1984;38:594-602.

44. Stallard P, Lenton S. How satisfied are parents of pre-school children who have special needs with the services they have received? A consumer survey. *Child: Care Health and Development.* 1992;18:197-205.

45. Law M, Dunn W. Perspectives on understanding and changing the environments of children with disabilities. *Phys Occup Ther Pediatr.* 1993;13(3):1-17.

46. Magrab PR, Schmidt LM. Interdisciplinary collaboration: a prelude to coordinated service delivery. In: Elder JO, Magrab PR, eds. *Coordinating Services to Handicapped Children: A Handbook for Interagency Cooperation*. Baltimore, MD: Paul H. Brookes; 1980: 13-23.

47. Francis D, Young D. *Improving Work Groups: A Practical Manual for Team Building*. San Diego, CA: University Associates; 1979.

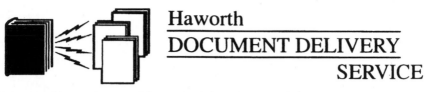

Haworth
DOCUMENT DELIVERY
SERVICE

This valuable service provides a single-article order form for any article from a Haworth journal.

- *Time Saving:* No running around from library to library to find a specific article.
- *Cost Effective:* All costs are kept down to a minimum.
- *Fast Delivery:* Choose from several options, including same-day FAX.
- *No Copyright Hassles:* You will be supplied by the original publisher.
- *Easy Payment:* Choose from several easy payment methods.

Open Accounts Welcome for . . .
- Library Interlibrary Loan Departments
- Library Network/Consortia Wishing to Provide Single-Article Services
- Indexing/Abstracting Services with Single Article Provision Services
- Document Provision Brokers and Freelance Information Service Providers

---

MAIL or *FAX* THIS ENTIRE ORDER FORM TO:

Haworth Document Delivery Service	**or FAX:** 1-800-895-0582
The Haworth Press, Inc.	**or CALL:** 1-800-342-9678
10 Alice Street	9am-5pm EST
Binghamton, NY 13904-1580	

PLEASE SEND ME PHOTOCOPIES OF THE FOLLOWING SINGLE ARTICLES:

1) Journal Title: _____
   Vol/Issue/Year: _____ Starting & Ending Pages: _____
   Article Title: _____
_____

2) Journal Title: _____
   Vol/Issue/Year: _____ Starting & Ending Pages: _____
   Article Title: _____
_____

3) Journal Title: _____
   Vol/Issue/Year: _____ Starting & Ending Pages: _____
   Article Title: _____
_____

4) Journal Title: _____
   Vol/Issue/Year: _____ Starting & Ending Pages: _____
   Article Title: _____
_____

(See other side for Costs and Payment Information)

COSTS: Please figure your cost to order quality copies of an article.

1. Set-up charge per article: $8.00
   ($8.00 × number of separate articles) _____

2. Photocopying charge for each article:

   1-10 pages: $1.00 _____

   11-19 pages: $3.00 _____

   20-29 pages: $5.00 _____

   30+ pages: $2.00/10 pages _____

3. Flexicover (optional): $2.00/article _____

4. Postage & Handling: US: $1.00 for the first article/
   $.50 each additional article _____

   Federal Express: $25.00 _____

   Outside US: $2.00 for first article/
   $.50 each additional article _____

5. Same-day FAX service: $.35 per page _____

   GRAND TOTAL: _____

METHOD OF PAYMENT: (please check one)

❑ Check enclosed   ❑ Please ship and bill. PO # _____
(sorry we can ship and bill to bookstores only! All others must pre-pay)

❑ Charge to my credit card: ❑ Visa; ❑ MasterCard; ❑ Discover;
❑ American Express;

Account Number: _____ Expiration date: _____

Signature: ✗ _____

Name: _____ Institution: _____

Address: _____

_____

City: _____ State: _____ Zip: _____

Phone Number: _____ FAX Number: _____

MAIL or *FAX* THIS ENTIRE ORDER FORM TO:

Haworth Document Delivery Service
The Haworth Press, Inc.
10 Alice Street
Binghamton, NY 13904-1580

or FAX: 1-800-895-0582
or CALL: 1-800-342-9678
9am-5pm EST)